Education for health

A manual on health education in primary health care

World Health Organization
Geneva
1988

Reprinted 1990

ISBN 92 4 154225 X

© World Health Organization 1988

TYPESET IN INDIA
PRINTED IN ENGLAND

87/7259—Macmillans/JB—8000

90/8445−JB−5000(R)

Contents

Chapter 4

Health education with individuals

Chapter 5

Health education with groups

Chapter 6

Health education with communities

Chapter 7
Communicating the health message: methods and media

Acknowledgements

The first version of this manual was prepared under a contract between the World Health Organization and the African Regional Health Education Centre, University of Ibadan, Nigeria. Under the direction of the Head of Department, Professor A.B.O.O. Oyediran, three staff members wrote the original document: Dr J. D. Adeniyi, W. R. Brieger, and B. E. Bassy, with graphic art provided by S. Iyi Ojediran. This was pre-tested with the family visitors, field overseers, and community nursing staff at the Igbo-Ora Rural Health Centre, Ibarapa Project, University of Ibadan.

The World Health Organization circulated over 100 copies of the original draft throughout the world for comment in 1980. Upon receipt of these comments, the services of W. R. Brieger as writer, A. Kaplun as editor, and G. Auberson as graphic artist were obtained, to produce a revised version of the manual. The World Heath Organization produced and circulated 7000 copies of a provisional version of the manual in 1984.

With feedback from the provisional version, W. R. Brieger and H. D. Ogden made final modifications to the text.

The John J. Sparkman Center for International Public Health Education, Birmingham, Alabama, USA, is associated with the publication of this manual as part of its agreement for collaborative cooperation with the World Health Organization.

A message from the Director-General of the World Health Organization[1]

World health will improve only if the people themselves become involved in planning, implementing, and having a say about their own health and health care. But involvement will not just happen.

How serious are we about involving individuals, families, and communities? Are we prepared—mentally and professionally—to listen to their concerns, to learn from them what they feel is important, to share with them appropriate information, to encourage and support them? Are we ready to assist them in choosing from alternative solutions, in setting their own targets and evaluating their efforts?

In many cases, so far, the answer is 'No'. We can go on and on developing plans: nothing will happen unless all health workers, all health managers, and key professionals in other sectors come to realize what is at stake.

To overcome these particular stumbling blocks, I see three major requirements.

First, health workers must understand that the concept of primary health care involves new roles for them, and a new outlook. Not only should we be concerned with disease prevention and control, we must also be concerned with health promotion and care. And not least with development in general—and with people. Our health technologies must be based on what the people themselves want and need. In other words, the health worker should learn first and foremost to act as a 'facilitator' of action by individuals, families, and communities. We must stop trying to fit communities into systems and programmes that we devise without a real and deep feeling for the social aspects of health problems or the economic constraints—not to speak of the cultural dissonance that is often the backlash of such programmes.

Second, health workers must accept their new roles. More yet: they must be keen to 'try them out', to adapt them, to broaden their scope and innovate in the partnership approach. Their main

[1]This text first appeared in the 1984 inaugural issue of *Education for health*, a newsletter issued by the World Health Organization in collaboration with the John J. Sparkman Center for International Public Health Education, Birmingham, Alabama, USA.

concern must be to find ways of helping individuals and communities become self-reliant. It must be made clear that advocating self-reliance in health matters in no way means abdicating our responsibilities and passing them on to others. Both lay persons and professionals are essential. They cannot replace each other, but they must work together.

This brings me to my third point: health workers must have the necessary skills to perform these new roles effectively and to make efficient use of existing knowledge. This calls for a training force fully familiar with accumulated experience, and keen to provide the kind and quality of professional preparation needed. It also calls for full backing from health managers for such training.

H. Mahler
Director-General
World Health Organization

Introduction

The goal to which WHO and all its Member States are pledged is 'Health for All by the Year 2000'. This inspiring goal can be attained only if health workers and the people themselves work effectively together.

Primary health care has been identified as the means of attaining this goal. Primary health care seeks to meet the essential health needs of as many people as possible, at the lowest possible cost. It includes the work of health centres, clinics, dispensaries, and doctors' offices in communities and neighbourhoods. But it also includes what individuals and families can do for themselves.

It is in this context that education and communication for health are especially important. For the truth is that individuals and families—not doctors and other health workers—make most of the important decisions that affect their health. Mothers decide what food to give their families and how to prepare it. Families decide when to go to a doctor or clinic, where to go, and whether or not to follow the instructions they receive from a health worker.

If these millions of daily decisions are to be made wisely, people need to be equipped with the knowledge and skills necessary to exercise individual and community responsibility. Primary health care is therefore very much concerned with health promotion and education.

To achieve effective participation by the community and individuals, two things need to be done.

Governments need to facilitate more community involvment in decision-making.

People need to be informed of their potential for improving their health through their own efforts.

The first—the governmental decision—is initially a political issue, but once the government decides to commit itself to community participation in health and development, it becomes a communications issue. 'All' in 'Health for All' means 'everybody'. In almost every country, there are media that can reach the whole population—everybody—with the message that they have an opportunity and a duty, as a matter of national policy, to contribute to their own health. People need to learn that their government is asking for their help in health improvement.

The second is basically an educational issue. People need to know how to carry out this mandate for their own benefit. This involves the adoption of certain types of behaviour and styles of living beneficial to health in individuals, families, neighbourhoods, and communities. It also involves educational assistance in building up more effective ways of organizing measures at the local level to identify and tackle local health problems.

As already suggested, major objectives of education for health are to enable people:

- to define their own problems and needs

- to understand what they can do about these problems with their own resources combined with outside support

- to decide on the most appropriate action to promote healthy living and community well-being.

Using this manual

Health education is central to primary health care, which in turn is the primary means of achieving 'Health for All'. Therefore, health education is a vital duty of health and other community workers who take part in primary health care.

This book is mainly addressed to such workers, in both urban and rural communities. It provides guidelines and ideas that public health officers, community nurses, agricultural extension workers, and other people who carry out education for health can adapt for use in their communities.

It is designed also to help them develop training programmes and technical support for community health workers. In this way the appropriate skills and techniques can be passed on to men and women who can use them in their community efforts.

Finally it is hoped that this manual will illustrate the link between health education efforts and communication at all levels, from the national to the local. National expressions of commitment to 'Health for All' can help to establish a climate that will encourage people in urban neighbourhoods and rural villages to work together for health. The community worker can take advantage of this spirit to advance specific projects.

This guide is specifically intended to help the reader:

- to integrate effective learning methods and approaches into the planning, delivery, and evaluation of primary health care services

- to design, carry out, and evaluate health activities, working with groups and individuals and using methods appropriate to the local culture and based on available resources

- to transfer educational and planning skills to community health workers and the community at large

- to promote effective interaction between person-to-person education at community level and communication to larger audiences through media of a local, regional, or national nature.

Health education focuses on people's ways of life and behaviour. In this manual:

- Chapter 1 explores the relationship between health and the behaviour of individuals, groups, and communities. It shows the importance of understanding the many reasons for people's behaviour.

- Chapter 2 deals with health education as 'people working with people', establishing good relationships, avoiding prejudice, knowing how to communicate clearly and how to promote partnership with people in achieving their goals.

- Chapter 3 reviews the skills needed for planning community health action. Such skills include collecting information, deciding on priorities, setting objectives, taking action, and evaluating results.

- Chapter 4 deals with health education as a process of counselling for individuals and families.

- Chapter 5 explores methods for the health education of groups, including formal and informal community groups, children at school, people in the same work-place, and the health care team itself. Methods for training groups are also included.

- Chapter 6 discusses techniques and approaches for working with the community as a whole.

- Finally, Chapter 7 describes various health education methods and media that can be used to promote wiser decision-making and improved health behaviour. It deals with person-to-person methods, with use of mass media, and with the effective combination of these approaches.

The concept of primary health care

The primary health care concept incorporates certain fundamental values common to the overall process of development but with emphasis on their application in the field of health, as follows:

- Health is fundamentally related to the availability and distribution of resources—not just health resources such as doctors, nurses, clinics, medicines, but also other socio-economic resources such as education, water and food supply.

- Primary health care is thus concerned with ensuring that the available health and social resources are distributed equitably, with due consideration for those whose needs are greatest.

- Health is an integral part of overall development. The factors influencing health are thus social, cultural, and economic, as well as biological and environmental.

- The achievement of better health requires much more involvement by people, as individuals, families, and communities, in taking action on their own behalf by adopting healthy behaviour and ensuring a healthy environment.

Primary health care is the first level of contact of individuals, the family and community with the national health system bringing health care as close as possible to where people live and work, and constitutes the first element of a continuing health care process.

Primary health care is the key to the attainment by all peoples of the world by the year 2000 of a level of health that will permit them to lead a socially and economically productive life.

Declaration of Alma-Ata, 1978

Chapter 1

Health behaviour and
health education

We have to think of many things when we want to help individuals, families, and communities prevent disease and promote health.

Spreading the word about what people should do to be healthy is important. But this is not enough. We have to understand that, in many situations, it is not only the individual who needs to change. There are other things that influence the way people behave: the place in which they live, the people around them, the work they do, whether they are able to earn enough money—all these things have a great influence, and we must take them into consideration.

Our first effort must be therefore to listen, to learn, and to understand.

In this chapter we will see:

- The factors that influence health and illness including people's own actions (pages 3–6).

- What makes people behave as they do (pages 6–15).

- Changes occurring in behaviour, naturally or through planned action (pages 15–18).

- Ways to help people improve their behaviour (pages 18–21).

Then we will discuss:

- What we really mean by health education (pages 22–24).

- Who is a health educator (pages 24–26).

Health, illness, and behaviour

An important background to health work is knowledge of what makes, and keeps, people healthy and why they become ill.[1]

---

[1] See also: *The community health worker.* Geneva, World Health Organization, 1987.

Dangers to health

A basic training in health tells us that many things, such as those listed below, are dangerous to health. You can probably think of more.

Living things

Tiny organisms such as bacteria, viruses, fungi, worms, and amoebae may enter the body through contact (touch), swallowing, and breathing, or through the bites and scratches of insects and other living things, and cause disease.

The bites and stings of animals such as scorpions and some snakes, bees, jellyfish, and spiders are dangerous to health.

Eating or touching certain plants can cause poisoning or rashes.

Non-living substances

Touching, swallowing or breathing substances such as kerosene, insecticides, gas, fertilizers, lead, and acid can poison or damage the body.

Alcohol, cigarettes, drugs used for non-medical reasons, like marijuana, and even medicines (if not taken correctly) can cause mental and physical illnesses.

Natural events

Floods, earthquakes, wind-storms, and similar events can cause injury and death.

In the natural process of growing older the human body becomes weaker and is more likely to suffer from illnesses.

Man-made environmental factors

Unguarded cooking fires, overcrowded houses, open gutters, broken bottles, open knife-blades, and poorly constructed roads and buildings can lead to accidents.

Stressful and difficult conditions at work, in the family, and in the community can lead to mental and physical illness.

Heredity

Certain diseases such as sickle cell anaemia, diabetes, and some forms of mental retardation can be inherited. The disease characteristic is passed on from mother, father, or both parents to the child.

The things listed on page 2 can certainly cause disease or injury, but alone they are not enough to do so. When there are open fires, bacteria, kerosene, or other dangerous things in the environment, people are not always injured, and do not always become ill. If people know how to deal with these dangerous things, trouble can be avoided.

Healthy and unhealthy behaviour

People stay healthy or become ill, often as a result of their own action or behaviour.

Here are some examples of how people's actions can keep them healthy:

- Washing hands and plates with soap and clean water kills some of the bacteria that cause disease.

- Using mosquito nets and insect sprays helps to keep disease-carrying mosquitos away.

- Putting kerosene bottles out of the reach of small children avoids the danger of children drinking from them and poisoning themselves.

- Carefully guarding cooking fires from children reduces the risk of burns.

In health education it is very important to be able to identify the practices that cause, cure, or prevent a problem. Let us look at a common health problem and see what kinds of behaviour are involved.

Diarrhoea is a common symptom of many diseases that are often the result of poor sanitation. It is a serious problem, especially in young children.

Here are some of the practices that can cause diarrhoea:

- Feeding children with feeding-bottles, as these are often difficult to keep clean.

- Drinking river, stream, or pond water without purifying it.

- Not washing hands before eating.

- Not washing plates, cups, and spoons, or washing them with plain water only.

3

- Defecating anywhere on the open ground. Infected faeces may contaminate objects that small children pick up and put in their mouths.

- Leaving refuse in the open, so flies can breed on it.

- Leaving food uncovered so that flies can contaminate it.

- Eating raw fruits and vegetables without washing them.

- Cooking food only partly, so that not all germs are killed.

- Using left-over food that has not been thoroughly reheated or that has spoiled.

Here are the kinds of action that can help control diarrhoea in a sick child:

- Giving the child plenty of liquids such as fruit juice and clean water.

- Continuing breast-feeding, rather than changing to a bottle, for children who are not completely weaned.

- Giving the child an oral rehydration drink made from clean water, salt, and sugar (check at your local clinic the formula that is accepted for use in your own country).

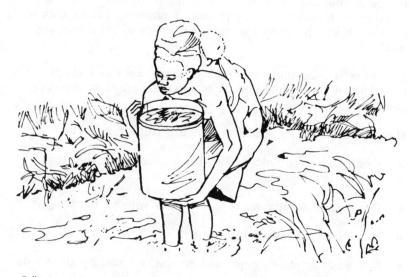

Collecting and drinking water from a pond like this one can help spread disease.

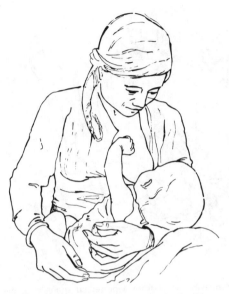

Breast-feeding of babies promotes health.

- Continuing feeding nutritious foods that will not upset the child's stomach (for example, avoid peppery foods).

- Going to the health worker the next day if the diarrhoea is not stopped by the simple actions just mentioned.

The following practices help prevent diarrhoea:

- Breast-feeding all infants.

- Filtering or boiling drinking-water from streams.

- Collecting drinking-water from sanitary wells or protected springs.

- Washing hands with soap and water before and after eating.

- Washing plates, cups, and spoons with clean water and soap.

- Defecating in latrines, and always washing hands with soap and water afterwards.

- Covering food to protect it from dust, insects, and other animals.

- Putting waste in a dustbin or a pit covered with soil, or burning it.

5

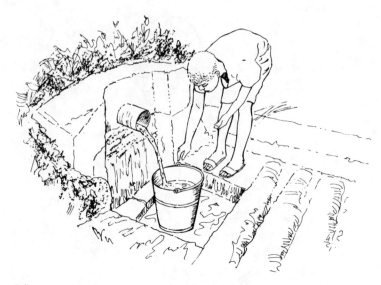

Collecting and drinking water from a protected spring is a means of promoting health. It is still necessary for the water to be collected in a clean bucket and stored in a clean container.

- Washing all food items.

- Washing hands with soap and water before preparing food.

- Cooking vegetables in boiling water.

Can you think of any other practices or kinds of behaviour that cause, control, or prevent diarrhoea?

Think of other health problems. What kind of behaviour can cause you to get a splinter in your foot? What kind of behaviour can prevent this? What kind of behaviour helps spread scabies? What kind of behaviour prevents it? Look at other common health problems in your area. Name the kinds of behaviour that cause, cure, and prevent them.

Understanding behaviour

There are many reasons why people behave the way they do. If we want to use health education to encourage healthy ways of life, we must know the reasons behind behaviour that causes or prevents illness. This knowledge will help us select the right educational methods for the problem at hand. Four main reasons for people's behaviour are given below.

Thoughts and feelings

We have many kinds of thoughts and feelings about the world we live in. These are shaped by our knowledge, beliefs, attitudes, and values, and they can help us decide whether to behave in one way or in another.

Knowledge

Knowledge often comes from experience. We also gain knowledge through information provided by teachers, parents, friends, books, and newspapers. We can usually verify whether our knowledge is correct or not. If we cannot verify this directly ourselves, we know people who can. The child who puts a hand in the cooking-fire gains knowledge about heat and pain. That knowledge stops the child doing the same thing again. A child may see a hen cross the road and be hit by a vehicle. From that experience the child should learn that the road can be dangerous, and to be more careful when crossing.

Beliefs

These are usually derived from our parents, grandparents, and other people we respect. We accept beliefs, without trying to prove that they are true. For example, in many countries there are beliefs regarding which foods a pregnant woman should and should not eat. In one country people believe that a pregnant woman must avoid eating certain meats: if not, her baby will behave like the animals from which the meat comes. These beliefs discourage pregnant women from eating certain foods. Think of other examples.

Every country and community has its own beliefs. In one country people believe that if a pregnant woman eats eggs, she will have a difficult delivery. But in another country people believe that a pregnant woman must eat eggs so that her baby will be strong and healthy. Beliefs are part of the way people live. They indicate what is acceptable and what is not. As beliefs can be held very strongly, they are often difficult to change. Sometimes health workers themselves believe that any traditional belief is bad and must be changed. This is not necessarily right. First, health workers should find out if the belief is harmful, helpful, or neutral. Once you understand how the belief affects people's health, then you can concentrate on trying to change only the harmful beliefs.

The belief that pregnant women should not eat eggs looks like a *harmful* one because eggs are a good source of protein, and. the mother needs to produce a strong and healthy baby. Before making a judgement about changing this belief, one should find out if the mothers in question are allowed to eat other good sources of protein such as meat, fish, beans, cheese, and groundnuts. If they get plenty of protein from other foods, it is not necessary to worry too much about the belief concerning eggs.

In one country there is a belief that, if a pregnant woman walks in the hot sun in the middle of the day, evil spirits will enter her body and damage the unborn child. One may not think that this belief is true. But it is sensible to encourage pregnant women not to overwork themselves when it is too sunny and hot. This type of belief may actually be *helpful*.

In many countries mothers put beads and charms on their children. They believe these beads will help the child. Some beads are believed to make teething easier, some to prevent illness, and others to protect against evil eye. One may doubt these beliefs. At the same time it is difficult to see any danger in the beads. Belief in their powers is probably a *neutral* belief, doing neither good nor harm.

If it is not certain that a belief is harmful, it is better to leave it alone. If too many of their beliefs are challenged people may get angry and not cooperate with the health workers.

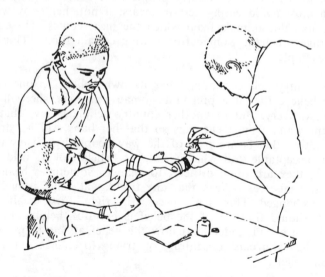

This child is wearing a lot of bracelets and beads. The mother believes that some of these bracelets will protect the child from disease. This belief does not stop the mother from consulting the health worker when the child is sick. It is a neutral belief, neither helping nor hurting. It is not necessary to change such a belief.

If we study people's beliefs carefully, we may even find ways of making them *useful*. For example, one health worker found it possible to tell if children were growing or losing weight by observing the beads they wore. The beads around a growing child's arm would be tight. The beads would hang loosely if the child was losing weight.

Make a list of the beliefs people in your community have about food. Which of these are harmful, helpful, or neutral? What do people in your village believe is the cause of fever? Which of these beliefs are harmful, helpful, or neutral? In some cases you may not be able to tell whether a belief is helpful, harmful, or neutral. In this case you must study the belief more carefully until you are certain of its effect on health.

Attitudes

These reflect our likes and dislikes. They often come from our experiences or from those of people close to us. They either attract us to things, or make us wary of them. Here is an example.

Mrs Mendoza's baby had a mild cold, so she took the baby to the health centre. The staff on duty that day were very busy and shouted at Mrs Mendoza 'Do you want us to waste our time over a simple cold? Come back when we are less busy.'

Mrs Mendoza did not like being shouted at. This experience gave her a bad attitude toward the health staff. She does not like or respect them now. This bad attitude could discourage Mrs Mendoza from attending the health centre next time her child is sick. However, an attitude about one thing alone does not always change how a person will behave. Mrs Mendoza may feel strongly that the drugs given at the health centre are very effective. Because of her attitude toward the drugs, Mrs Mendoza may still go to the health centre for help even though she still has a bad attitude towards the staff.

Attitudes can also come from other people's experiences.

Mrs Toro, for example, remembered that her neighbour's baby was successfully treated at the health centre. The positive attitude towards the health centre, which Mrs Toro had gained from her neighbour's experience, encouraged her to go to the health centre next time her own baby was sick.

On the other hand, situations do not always allow us to behave according to our attitudes. Maybe Mrs Toro is afraid of the dark, or possibly the health centre might be closed at night. If the baby fell sick at night, she might go to the old grandmother next door instead of walking to the centre in the dark. This does not mean her attitude towards the health centre has changed.

Attitudes are sometimes based on limited experience. We may form attitudes without understanding the whole situation. For example:

> Mr Nola had bad results from a packet of seeds he bought in the town. From his experience with only one packet, he formed the attitude that the shopkeeper who sold the seeds was a bad person. Because of this attitude, Mr Nola decided never to go to that person's shop again.

There are many possible reasons why the seeds grew poorly. It was not correct to blame the shopkeeper without looking into the situation more deeply.

Think about your own attitudes. Take, as an example, sprays for killing insects. You may have seen many different sprays: which do you think are good? Which is the best? Why do you have these attitudes about these sprays? How do these attitudes affect your behaviour? Do you always buy the spray you feel is best? If not, why not?

Values

These are the beliefs and standards that are most important to us. People in a community share many values. For example they may want their community to be stable and happy. One way to work towards these values is by cooperation. Cooperation means working together to solve problems. It makes life easier. For example, in a community that values stability and happiness if one family wants to build a new house, the other villagers will cooperate together and help with the building.

The welfare of children is another value. By taking good care of children, parents will benefit: when healthy children grow up, they will be able to take care of their parents in old age. The value attached to children may encourage a mother to stay at home and care for a sick child instead of going out to visit her friends.

Think about your own values. What are the things that are most important in your life? How do these values affect your own behaviour? Think about the values of the community where you work. What values do you share with these people? Are any of your values different from theirs? How do the community's values encourage people to behave towards each other and with regard to health?

People who are important to us

A second reason for our behaviour is the influence of people who are very important to us. When someone is important to us, we often listen to what he or she says and try to do what he or she does.

Among these important people are parents, grandparents, village leaders, religious leaders, close friends, workmates, people with a lot of experience and special skills, and people who try to help us when we need it (teachers, health workers, social workers).

Schoolteachers are very important to their pupils. If pupils see teachers washing their hands before eating, they may copy this behaviour.

Everyone likes to have friends. Because they are important to us, we often copy their behaviour. If a teenage boy has close friends who smoke cigarettes, he may start to smoke too.

Mr Tome is an old, experienced farmer. When he tells the other farmers not to plant their crops until they see the new moon after the first rain, they will follow his advice. Even if the agricultural agent gives them different advice, these farmers may tend to respect and copy the actions of the old man. They may not want to listen to a young extension agent who, in addition, may come from a different town.

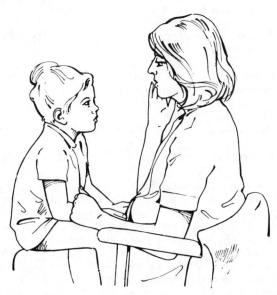

A mother is an important person to her child. The words and actions of the mother are likely to influence the behaviour of the child.

Who are the respected people in your family? Who are the important and respected people in your village? What kinds of behaviour do these important people encourage in your family and in the community?

Resources

A third reason for people's behaviour is whether or not they have certain resources. Resources include facilities, money, time, labour, services, skills, and materials. The location of material resources is also important. If a resource is found a long way from the community it may not be used. Having a lot of things to do in a short time often affects people's behaviour. For example:

Time

Time is a valuable resource.

Mr Aba is a tailor. He has a lot of work to do because a holiday is coming soon. If he cannot deliver orders on time, his customers will get angry and may go to another tailor next time. But Mr Aba has a headache and catarrh today. His wife suggests that he goes to the health centre for help. He tells her 'The health centre is always crowded. If I go there, I will waste too much time. I shall go to the drug-seller and buy my own medicines.'

Time has affected Mr Aba's behaviour. The health service is an important resource but it may not be useful if it is too crowded.

Money

Money is needed for some kinds of behaviour. For example:

Mrs Ebra has four children. Her husband died last year in an accident. She does not have a trade and has no particular *skill* (another important resource). She collects and sells firewood to make money to feed her children. The health worker tells Mrs Ebra that she should give her children meat, eggs, and milk to make them strong. Mrs Ebra says that she cannot afford these expensive things. The health worker has to think carefully. What can Mrs Ebra buy with her few resources? Finally, they agree that beans and rice can be afforded, with some fish added once or twice a week. Then the health worker sends Mrs Ebra to the social development worker to see about training in a skill that will help her to earn more money.

Some people carry on doing dangerous work because of money, or for cultural reasons. For example the man in the illustration is a palm-wine tapper. He runs the risk of falling and injuring himself or of suffering from back pains. He may carry on doing this work for several reasons. Perhaps his father did the same kind of work, and influenced him to continue in the same line; or perhaps he believes there is a spirit protecting him from injury; or this may be the only job he can find to earn money for his family.

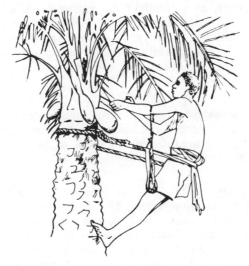

This man is a palm-wine tapper.

Drinking water directly from a stream is a behaviour that causes many diseases. A hygienic well is a *facility* that prevents those diseases.

The people in Pembo village want a well in order to reduce the number of illnesses they suffer from. They first need the *skills* that will enable them to find a place for a well that will have enough water. They ask their health worker to contact the right ministry or agency and request an expert to help them find a good place for the well. Next the villagers need *materials*, such as cement and shovels, for which they may also need to raise *money*. The people are willing to contribute their *labour* for digging the well. When the expert comes he shows them several places in which they could dig the well. They choose the place closest to the village, as they know that if the distance to the well is too great people may not want to use it.

These are some of the resources the people of Pembo need in order to change their behaviour and begin drinking clean water. Can you think of others?

Culture

Most of the issues presented in the previous sections vary from one community to another. The normal forms of behaviour, beliefs, values, and use of resources in a community form a pattern or way of life. This is known as culture. Cultures have been developed over many hundreds or thousands of years by people living together and sharing experiences in a certain environment. Cultures continue to change, sometimes slowly, sometimes quickly, as a result of natural or social events or contact with people of other cultures. What is important here is to note that culture or life-style is a combination of most of what has just been discussed. While normal behaviour is one of the aspects of a culture, culture in its turn has a deep influence on behaviour.

In a practical sense, you can see, hear, and understand culture whenever you are in the community by observing people's dress, common foods, and organization of work or by listening to songs, proverbs, fables, and ordinary speech.

Greetings vary among cultures—an embrace, a handshake, a kiss, special words, to mention a few. The way people eat is part of culture: with wooden sticks, with fingers, or with metal cutlery; in family groups, groups of children, or groups of men only; sitting on chairs, mats, or benches. There are many possibilities. Each culture has its own special way of doing things, and beliefs about why things should be done in that way.

This common pattern of behaviour, beliefs, and values helps people understand and feel comfortable with life. Each culture represents one way that people have found for living together in their environment. When people come to a new community and culture, they are unsettled at first because they do not know what behaviour and ideas are acceptable. Health workers, teachers, and other community workers are often in this situation. Their training has made them part of a 'professional' culture. They have their own ideas and ways of doing things, which are often quite different from those of the community. Before they begin their work, they should learn as much as possible about the reasons for people's behaviour in the community. This will help them to work in an acceptable way with the community they wish to serve.

As we have seen, there are many reasons for people's behaviour. It is even possible that different people or communities may behave in the same ways but for very different reasons, as the following examples show.

Three mothers may all give fruit to their children. When you ask why, they give different answers.

Mrs Gomez says, 'I believe that if my children eat fruit they will be healthier.'

Mrs Paulo says, 'My mother-in-law lives with us. She said that she always gave my husband fruit when he was small, so I must give fruit to my own children.'

Mrs Andre says, 'I prefer to buy fruit for my children. It costs less than sweets and snacks'.

There may be concern about the safety of the water in your community. When you visit the different neighbourhoods, you find that three of them have wells but for different reasons.

People in the first neighbourhood tell you, 'We dug our well because we learned that well-water is cleaner than stream-water.'

In the second neighbourhood you hear, 'We saw that the leading people in town had wells, so we decided to build our own.'

Residents of the third neighbourhood say, 'We used to collect water from a far-away stream. That wasted time and energy. We built a well to make life easier.'

By knowing something about the possible reasons for a given form of behaviour, you will be able to suggest appropriate changes and solutions to the problems you have noticed. Now look at your own community. What are the eating habits of the people? What are some of the reasons for people eating one food and not another? How do people dispose of refuse in your village? Why do they do it that way? How do people in your area keep their mouths and teeth clean? What are the reasons for these ways of behaving? How can you find out about the reasons?

Changes in behaviour

In all communities there are already many kinds of behaviour that promote health, prevent illness, and help in the cure and rehabilitation of sick people. These kinds of behaviour should be identified and encouraged. In fact it is usually the positive, healthy results of such behaviours that encourage people to continue with them.

There is also behaviour that is harmful to health. Because of the unhealthy results of such behaviour, people often give it up by themselves. Sometimes, for the reasons mentioned in the previous sections, people go on behaving in an unhealthy way.

Before beginning a health education activity, it is necessary to have an understanding of the difficulties people often face when trying to make improvements in their lives. This understanding will help in the selection of appropriate health education methods.

Natural change

Our behaviour changes all the time. Some changes take place because of natural events. When changes take place in the community around us, we often change ourselves without thinking much about it. This is natural change. Here are some examples.

Mrs M usually buys red beans at the market, but she may change her behaviour and buy white beans if no red ones are available.

Mr P wears a light shirt in the hot, dry season, but when cool, rainy weather comes, he may change to wearing a heavy shirt.

Mr R is a farmer. Normally he walks directly north to reach his fields, but, because of heavy rain and flooding, he changes his usual route and walks east first to find a better path.

Planned change

Sometimes we make plans to improve our lives. Here are some examples.

Mr G smokes many cigarettes each day. Now he has started coughing a lot. He decides he will stop smoking. He plans a date in a couple of weeks time when he will stop smoking, and starts to prepare himself for this.

Mrs H wants to buy some new clothes for her children. She usually spends her extra money on sweets and soft drinks. Now instead of buying sweets, she plans to save her money until she has enough to buy her children some clothes.

Mr J has been living in his father's house for many years. He now has a wife and three children. The father's house has become crowded, and it is old. Mr J plans to build a bigger house for his own family and his parents.

Now think about yourself. Have you made any changes in your own behaviour recently? What were these changes? Why did you make them?

Look at your community. Have there been any changes in the way the villagers behave? What are those changes? Why did those changes happen? How did they come about?

Readiness to change

You may know some people who are always quick to try something new. They buy the newest tools and seeds, they wear the latest style of clothes. Other people are very slow to change. Not everyone is ready to change at the same time. Here is a story about readiness to change.

A group of mothers were waiting at the preschool clinic. The midwife decided to talk to them about caring for their children's feet. This is because the midwife had seen so many small children with cuts, sores, and ulcers on their feet. The action the midwife asked the mothers to take was to buy shoes for their children.

Mrs Uba was sitting in the group. Her two-year-old daughter always ran about barefoot and had cuts and ulcers. This always made Mrs Uba worry. Today she learned that disease could enter the body through cuts. She had a good business selling cloth so she knew that she could afford the shoes. Her husband was always asking about the welfare of the child. He would support any action that would protect his daughter. Mrs Uba decided to buy shoes. She was ready to change. There were no serious problems to stop her.

Mrs Odom sat next to Mrs Uba. Her son did not have shoes either. Mrs Odom also accepted the information that dirty cuts on the foot could bring illness. She wanted to do the best for her child. Mrs Odom was working on the farm with her husband. Although they were poor, they were always thinking about how to help their children. Their grandmother lived with them. Mrs Odom knew that the grandmother would not approve of spending money on shoes. She would say 'My son never wore shoes until he was grown. Why should we buy shoes for this baby?' Mrs Odom was interested in changing but had to solve some other problems first.

Mrs Tembo sat at the back of the group. She did not like the midwife. The midwife had scolded her many times because her child was often sick. Although she knew that the midwife was giving sensible information, Mrs Tembo was not paying close attention because of her bad attitude to the midwife and because of the many other worries on her mind. Mrs Tembo's husband had run away after their baby was born. Now she managed to

17

make a little money doing washing for other people. Because of these problems, Mrs Tembo was hard to reach. Health information from this midwife was not enough to encourage Mrs Tembo to change.

At the beginning of the midwife's talk, none of these mothers had bought shoes for their children. What were the reasons for their behaviour? After the talk, only Mrs Uba followed the midwife's advice. Why was this? Why did the others not buy shoes? How could you help Mrs Odom and Mrs Tembo with their problems?

Helping people to lead healthier lives

It is natural for people to help each other. This is especially useful when people have to solve difficult problems. There are some people whose full-time job is helping others. Among them are teachers, social workers, policemen, agricultural agents, religious leaders, and, of course, health workers. There are three general ways in which these people can try to help other people lead healthier lives:

- They can force or push people to change, and threaten punishment if the changes are not made.

- They can give ideas or information in the hope that people will use them to improve their lives.

- They can meet with people to discuss problems and promote their interest and participation in choosing the best ways to solve their own problems.

Let us look at three examples of how a health worker can provide help.

Using force

There was once a family who did not keep their home and land clean. They would throw their rubbish and faeces onto a big pile just behind the house. This pile became a home for rats, flies, and mosquitos. It is not surprising that the children of this family often had fever and diarrhoea.

One day Mr D, a health worker, visited the family. He was very sad when he saw their home. He told the family that they were making trouble for themselves and for the whole community. They did not pay attention. He came again and again — with no result. Finally, he told the family that if they did not clean up the place by the next week, he would take them to court where they would have to pay a big fine. The family was afraid of this, so they quickly cleaned their house and yard.

The health worker came the next week, as promised. He saw that the place was clean. He then told the family that they must always keep the place clean. He again threatened to take them to court if they disobeyed him. The man left and did not come back for some months.

When the family had not seen the man for some time, they decided that his threat had not been serious and they became angry. They did not see why a stranger should come to their house and push them around. Soon they began throwing rubbish behind the house again.

Finally, the health worker returned and saw the mess. But this time when he tried to talk to the family they told him to go away. They said they would fight him if he tried to enter their house.

Thus when the health worker attempted to force and push the family, they did what he said at first; later they became angry and refused to cooperate.

Giving information

The season in which many children get measles was coming to Patel village. The health workers there were worried because not many of the children had been immunized against measles. They decided to call a meeting of the village leaders and mothers.

At the meeting the health workers talked all about measles. They said it was caused by a tiny virus that spread through the air from one child to another. This happened especially in places where children were close together. They explained that measles appears as a rash. There is also fever. The dangers of measles were listed as pneumonia, blindness, and death. The disease, they noted, spread more easily at that time of year, so the health workers asked all villagers to bring their children to the health centre on a Wednesday morning as soon as possible. At the centre a special injection would be given to protect or 'immunize' the children from the disease.

After about a month the health workers noticed that very few mothers had brought their children for the measles immunization. They became worried. They knew that they had given correct information to the villagers. They went to the village leaders to find out what was happening.

The village leaders told the health workers many things. First they said that the villagers believe measles is caused by the smoke from certain types of firewood. Secondly, they did not want to believe that the disease could pass· from one person to another. Finally, they said that some mothers wanted the immunization, but would have difficulty coming to the health centre, because the most important market in the area was held every Wednesday morning.

These health workers did better than the one in the first example. They did not use force. They got a few people to come for immunization. But they were not successful enough. Even though the health information they gave was correct, it was not enough to encourage most mothers to bring their children for immunization. There were other influences on the mothers' behaviour that the health worker had not taken into account.

Discussing and participating

Good health workers visit people in their community and listen to their problems.

One day Mrs M, a health worker, came to see a group of farmers. She sat and listened to their problems for a while. The farmers were complaining of being weak and tired. The health worker saw that they were very pale. She suspected that the farmers had hookworm.

First, the health worker asked the farmers what they thought caused their problem. Some said overwork. Others said the weather was too hot. One even said that farmers from the next village were jealous and were using magic to cause the weakness. Then the health worker asked what the farmers had been doing to solve the problem. One said his wife was making him eat more. Another said he was going to sleep early. A few said that they were drinking tonics made from herbs. The health worker asked if any of these actions had cured the problem. All of the farmers said 'No'.

Next, the farmers asked the health worker if she could help them. The health worker said that she would try but that she would need to know more about the farmers' daily work. She asked what the farmers wore at work. Their answer was 'Short trousers and a singlet or light shirt'. Did they wear anything on their feet? The answer was 'No'. Where did they defecate while on the farm? The farmers said that they eased themselves anywhere nearby.

The health worker said 'Thank you. Your answers give me some idea about the problem. Do you know that small worms can get inside people?' A few mentioned that they had seen worms in their stools occasionally. The worms must have got in somehow.

'There are different worms, with different ways of entering the body,' said the health worker. 'Once inside, some worms eat food in the gut while others eat blood, making people weak. One worm called hookworm gives farmers a lot of trouble because it is in the soil. It is possible that this worm might be causing your problem. After burrowing into someone's foot, it moves to the gut where it hooks on and drinks blood. The worms are not always seen in the stools.' 'When a person defecates, some of the tiny eggs of the worm pass with the stool,' added the health worker. Some farmers were not sure about this. One asked 'Why is hot weather not to blame?' The health worker replied that hot weather helps the eggs of the worm to hatch and grow in the soil. 'What about our jealous neighbours?' asked another farmer. The health worker explained that neighbours could spread hookworm by defecating in the fields although they may not know about hookworm either. Finally, the farmers accepted these ideas.

The health worker asked 'Now what can you do to prevent hookworm?' One farmer answered, 'Wear shoes.' The others did not like this idea because shoes were costly and hot. Another said, 'Use latrines'. The rest laughed, because they said they could not afford to build a latrine on every farm.

The health worker asked if there were more simple and less expensive things the farmers could do. One farmer said 'Sandals are cheap. Local shoemakers make them, and rubber and plastic ones are sold in the market.' Another farmer suggested 'We could use our hoes to dig a hole each time we defecate.' The group liked these ideas. They all agreed to buy sandals and to bury their faeces when on the farm. The health worker commented that burying faeces on the farm could be dangerous unless it was done far from any place where someone might dig it up by mistake when ploughing.

Before she left, the health worker asked all the farmers to meet her at the clinic. There she could test their faeces for worms and, if hookworm eggs were seen, she could give them medicine to kill the worms. She reminded them of the farmer's wife who had said that her husband should eat more. The health worker said that this was wise because the worms had eaten so much blood. She said that green leafy vegetables and meat would help make their blood strong again. Of course they should clean and cook the vegetables and meat well. The farmers thanked the health worker. The next day all the farmers came to the clinic. Every one of them was wearing sandals.

This health worker was successful. She did not push people and did not merely give information. She helped people think about their own problems and asked them to think about the ways of solving the problems. These farmers participated. In the end they all agreed to take the actions that would improve their health.

The role of health education

In the three examples just described, only one health worker was practising health education. It was the third health worker, who encouraged the people to understand their problems and choose the most appropriate solutions for themselves.

Think about the problems facing the first two health workers. What should those health workers have done if they had wanted to use health education?

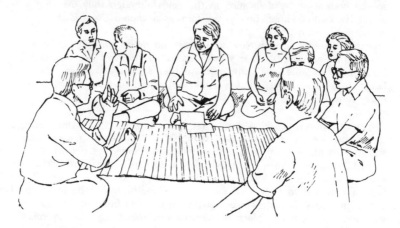

The health education approach encourages people to talk about their problems and to find their own solutions to them. The role of the health worker is to help people consider what solution is best.

Health workers can use health education successfully by:

- Talking to the people and listening to their problems.
- Thinking of the behaviour or action that could cause, cure, and prevent these problems.
- Finding reasons for people's behaviour (beliefs, friends' ideas, lack of money, and others).
- Helping people to see the reasons for their actions and health problems.
- Asking people to give their own ideas for solving the problems.
- Helping people to look at their ideas so that they could see which were the most useful and the simplest to put into practice.
- Encouraging people to choose the idea best suited to their circumstances.

What do we really mean by health education?

Health education is the part of health care that is concerned with promoting healthy behaviour.

A person's behaviour may be the main cause of a health problem, but it can also be the main solution. This is true for the teenager who smokes, the mother with the poorly nourished child, and the butcher who gets a cut on his finger. By changing their behaviour these individuals can solve and prevent many of their own problems.

Through health education we help people understand their behaviour and how it affects their health. We encourage people to make their own choices for a healthy life. We do not force people to change.

Health education does not replace other health services, but it is needed to promote the proper use of these services. One example of this is immunization: scientists have made many vaccines to prevent diseases, but this achievement is of no value unless people go to receive the immunization. Similarly, incinerators for burning refuse are useless unless people will make the effort to put the refuse inside the incinerators.

Health education encourages behaviour that promotes health, prevents illness, cures disease, and facilitates rehabilitation. The needs and interests of individuals, families, groups, organizations, and communities are at the heart of health education programmes. Thus there are many opportunities for practising health education.

Health education is not the same thing as health information. Correct information is certainly a basic part of health education, but health education must also address the other factors that affect health behaviour such as availability of resources, effectiveness of community leadership, social support from family members, and levels of self-help skills. Health education therefore uses a variety of methods to help people understand their own situations and choose actions that will improve their health. Health education is incomplete unless it encourages involvement and choice by the people themselves. For example merely telling people to follow "good health behaviour" is not health education. Although bringing a child monthly to the clinic for weighing is a behaviour that promotes health some mothers may see the situation differently. Some may believe that a child who is healthy does not need to attend a clinic. Some mothers may not see any purpose in weighing babies, and some may feel that their housework and other jobs are more important than weighing a healthy baby. In health education these different views are considered when seeking solutions to problems.

Also, in health education we do not blame people if they do not behave in a healthy way. Often unhealthy behaviour is not the

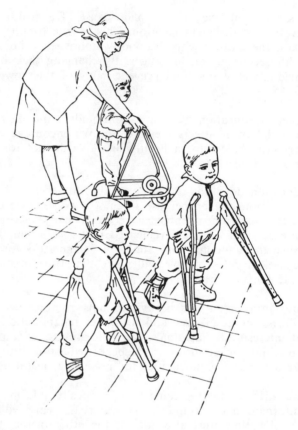

In additiion to preventing disease, health education can be used for many other purposes. As shown here, it can play a part in providing skills for the rehabilitation of handicapped people.

fault of the individual. In health education we must work with families, communities, and even regional and national authorities to make sure that resources and support are available to enable each individual to lead a healthy life.

Who is a health educator?

Once we understand what health education is about, it is important to answer the question, 'Who is a health educator?' It is true that some people are specially trained to do health education work. We may refer to those people as specialists. But since all health workers are concerned with helping people to improve their health knowledge and skills, all health workers should practise health education in their jobs. By carrying out health education activities, nurses, dispensers and, of course, community health workers, can make health care more effective.

Health education, then, is really the duty of everyone engaged in health and community development activities.

If health and other workers are not practising health education in their daily work, they are not doing their job correctly. When treating someone with a skin infection or malaria, a health worker should also educate the patient about the cause of the illness and teach preventive skills. Drugs alone will not solve problems. Without health education, the patient may fall sick again and again from the same disease.

Likewise, an environmental sanitation programme should include health education. It is not enough for the ministry or an agency to provide sanitary wells, latrines, and waste collection facilities: the people will continue to suffer from the diseases caused by poor sanitation if they do not use the facilities. If a health education approach is taken, the people will participate from the beginning in identifying their sanitation problems and will choose the solutions and facilities they want. They will then be more likely to use these facilities and improve their health.

Health workers must also realize that their own personal example serves to educate others. The midwife who does not wear a clean

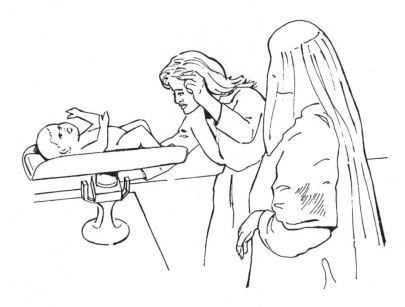

A healthy baby being weighed at a clinic.

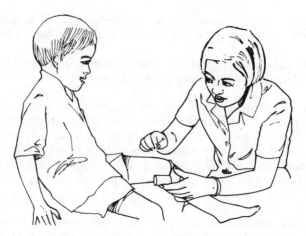

Health workers have many opportunities to practise health education while they are treating patients. For example explaining to a child why it is important to keep cuts clean, rather than just dressing the cut.

uniform and the dispenser who does not sweep his first-aid post clean set bad examples. People will not believe these health workers when they talk about health and hygiene. On the other hand, health workers who build latrines in their own houses, purify their drinking-water and feed their children nutritious food will, by example, teach their neighbours healthy habits.

Chapter 2

People working with people

In health education we are concerned about how people actually feel, not how we think they should feel. We are interested in how people look at their own problems, not only in the problems we see ourselves. We want people to develop the confidence and skills to help themselves. We do not look for thanks or praise, but we do aim at a feeling of pride in the fact that people have learned the skills needed to solve their own problems.

To enable people to learn these skills, we need:

● To establish good relationships (pages 27–29).

● To communicate clearly (pages 29–32).

● To encourage participation (pages 32–36).

● To avoid prejudice and bias (pages 36–38).

These are the four points examined in this chapter.

Establishing good relationships

Helping relationships

There are many people whose job is to help other people. For example, there are teachers, social welfare workers, extension agents, nurses, and others.

As a 'front-line' health worker, you also belong to the category of helping professionals. In order to be a successful helper, you must have a good relationship with those you want to help. If people like you, if they trust you, and if they feel comfortable with you, then you will be in a better position to help them.

You can get people to trust you by respecting them (regardless of who they are, what they believe, or where they come from), by listening to them, and by encouraging them to develop their own strengths.

The person you are

Who you are (your personality) and what you do (your actions) influence the way people look at you and think about you. Your personality and actions also influence the type of relationship you have with people in the community.

You are a health worker, but you are also many other things. You are a certain age and sex, you belong to a certain family, a social group, and a work group. You may be a member of a religious group. All these factors determine how the people in the community view you and what they expect of you. Different kinds of behaviour may be expected of people according to their age, sex, religion, or type of work.

Know about the community's expectations and be aware of your own personality. This will help you in developing good relations within your community. Learn about yourself and your personality by observing how others react to you. If you find that community members generally are not listening to you or are avoiding you, ask trusted friends or co-workers if they have also observed this. Ask if they know any possible reasons for such a reaction. From what you learn about yourself, try to change the aspects of your character that worry the community.

How to establish good relationships

If you are to establish good relationships, people must see you at work. You must be visible to them. You must do things that

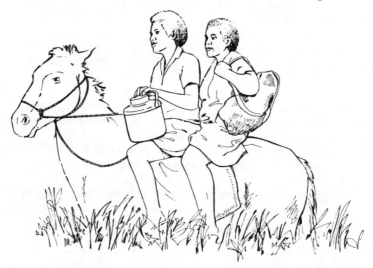

In order to establish a good relationship, it is necessary to visit the community often, using whatever means is available. These health workers travel by horse to reach the villages they serve. Others may use bicycles, motorcycles, public buses, or lorries, or they may walk.

people believe are useful and beneficial. You must reach out to people and explain your job to them. You must also listen to people and show concern about their problems and needs. You must always be available to give help when people need it.

When you start working in a community, you should introduce (or reintroduce) yourself to people in that community. Visit the leaders and representatives of all the various groups. Meet with the other people who work to improve the community. Visit religious and political leaders, teachers, agricultural workers, traditional healers, other health workers, and social welfare workers. Learn about their work. Explain your job to them. Discuss how all of you can work together to make your community better.

Finally, remember that the purpose of health education is to help people solve their problems by their own efforts. It is your role to help community members realize what they can do to help themselves, and to teach them the skills needed to do so. By using health education methods in your work, you will be able to help people to do something good about health. People will then feel better about themselves. They will also appreciate you for your concern and for your interest in their welfare. Your relationships will grow and improve.

Who are the people in your private or professional life you have good relationships with? What makes those relationships good? Are there any people you do not have such a good relationship with? What can you do to improve your relationships with those people?

Communicating clearly

Every day of our lives we try to share ideas, feelings, and information with other people. This is known as 'communication'. Talking is the most common way of communicating, but there are many others, for example: writing, making hand and body movements, drawing, singing, and so on. Many of the educational methods that we will discuss later are in fact communication methods. Communication skills are needed in health education.

Communication is part of our normal relationship with other people. A good relationship cannot exist without some sharing of ideas, feelings, and information. Likewise sharing happens most easily between people who have a good relationship. Building good relationships with people—as discussed in the previous section—goes hand in hand with developing communication skills. Three important skills needed for good communication are discussed below.

Talking and presenting clearly

The goal of communication is to make sure that people hear, see, and understand the message (idea or feeling) that is being shared with them. Therefore it is important to talk, write,. or present this message clearly and simply.

First, use words that people will understand. Many words relating to health care, such as immunization, disinfection, antiseptic, hypertension, and tuberculosis, will be unfamiliar to people. Find simple, common words to explain what is meant. For example, say 'make very clean' for disinfect. Find out the local names for diseases. A health worker who participates in community activities and knows about the local culture will be able to use words and ideas that are familiar to the people.

Another aspect of clear communication is using as few words as possible. A long lecture will bore people. They will miss or forget the message.

When educational methods based on materials such as posters, films, and photographs are used, it is necessary for people to be familiar with those methods. A method that is strange to people may not communicate the right idea. Make sure all words, written or spoken, used to educate people, are clear and simple.

Listening and giving attention

Communication involves both giving and receiving. Not only should the health worker speak clearly to the community, he or she must listen carefully to its members in order to understand their interests and ideas.

Listening is a way of showing respect. Pay close attention to what people tell you. Encourage them to speak freely. Do not stop them, interrupt them, or begin to argue. This will cut off communication, and you may get only half the message, or nothing at all.

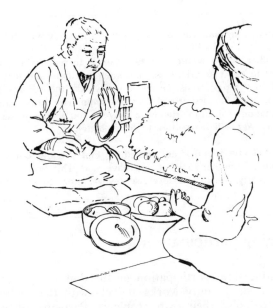

The art of listening is very important in health education. By listening carefully, the health worker learns how a person feels about a problem and the reasons for his or her behaviour. Then, it becomes possible to help the person find appropriate solutions.

While listening, do not look at something else. Do not busy yourself with work while the other person is talking. If you do these things, the other person will think you do not care about him or her.

Discussing and clarifying

After listening, it is important to make sure you have heard the other person correctly. Similarly, after talking, you should find out if the other person has heard you correctly. Asking questions can help clarify what someone said. Never be afraid to ask questions. Questions can make communication between people more accurate.

It is also good to summarize. After listening, try briefly to tell the other person what you think was said. Then ask the person if you have understood their ideas and meaning. Do the same when you do the talking: encourage the other person to summarize your words. Then you will know whether what you said was understood. This kind of discussion between people leads to good communication.

31

Here is something you can do to practise your communication skills.

Ask two other health workers or two friends to meet with you. Ask one friend to tell you briefly about something important that has happened in the past week. Listen carefully. Ask the second friend to listen also. After the first friend finishes, summarize briefly and repeat the information. Ask both friends to correct you if you made mistakes. In this way you will learn how to listen better.

Next you tell one friend about something that you did last week. Ask your friend to summarize what you have said. This way you will learn to speak clearly. Repeat this exercise several times to practise your skills.

Encouraging participation

In health education, participation means that the person, the group, or the community works actively with the health workers and others to solve their own problems. Participation is necessary at every step, from identifying problems to solving them. After you have established your relationship with people and communities, you should immediately begin to encourage participation. Use your communication skills and encourage people to talk while you listen. In that way they can participate in identifying their own problems.

Why should people participate? First, if people participate, they will be more interested in helping themselves. They will also be more committed to taking the action necessary to improve their health.

Second, people are responsible for their own health. Health workers can guide people in finding solutions to problems, but cannot take direct responsibility. If a mother arrives with a poorly fed baby, a health worker cannot take the baby home and feed it. If health workers give drugs to people to cure fever, they cannot follow the people home and put the tablets in their mouths every four hours. If a community complains that it does not have a good water supply, health workers cannot give the money for digging the well. Of course they can help, but the most important help is self-help. Health workers have many opportunities to encourage self-help. See the illustration on page 33 for an example.

Participation in identifying problems

Health workers make a mistake if they say to a community 'we know what your main problems are.' It is true that health

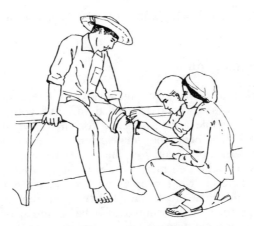

This community health worker is using health education to encourage self-help. While she is treating the husband, she is also teaching him and his wife the simple skills needed to care for the wound.

workers see many problems. They may look at clinic records and see that many people suffer from malaria. This is a problem. They may visit the community and see refuse scattered about. This is a problem, too. But, until the people concerned understand that there is a problem, they will not be interested in solving it. You may make people angry if you assume that you know all about their lives.

Encourage people to identify their own problems first, then they will be more ready to deal with them. Most of the problems will be related to health somehow. Health workers should show an interest in helping with the problems that the members of the community see. This will help build trust and strengthen relationships.

Participation in finding solutions

If health workers say 'we know the best solution to your problem', they are making another mistake. Things that are 'best' for one person or one community may not be so for another. Communities have different amounts of resources. They have different beliefs and values. They have different types of leaders. The solution for a problem must fit the real-life situation of the person or community. This can be done through the participation of the person or community concerned.

Of course a health worker can make suggestions, but ideas should come from the people first—the more ideas the better. Examine each suggestion carefully with the people concerned to see if it

33

will work. Then encourage people to select the solution that is best for them.

Participation in action

A health worker also makes a big mistake if he or she says 'Don't worry. I will do what is needed to solve your problem.' Remember that people are responsible for their own health. If you do all the work for them, they may criticize the results and blame you. But this does not mean you should let them do everything by themselves. On the contrary, be clear about what you can and should do, and about what people can do and learn to do for themselves. While there are certain health tasks that a trained person must perform, there should also be as much opportunity as possible for participation so that, through experience, community members will gain skills.

Facilitating participation

Remember to avoid the common mistakes mentioned above. Think about what 'we' can do to solve problems, not what 'I' can do. You are a guide and a helper.

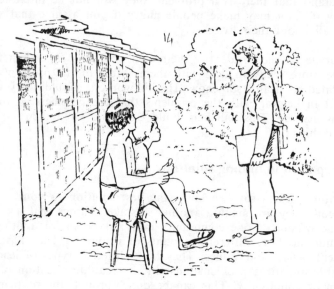

Don't worry. I will do what is needed to solve your problem.' This approach is likely to create more problems in the long run, rather than solve any. Why? Because people become dependent on the health worker. A major objective should be to help people become self-reliant and give them the skills that will enable them to participate actively at every step of primary health care from identifying problems to solving them.

Together with the people, you should ask 'What problems can we identify? What are the best solutions we can select? What action can we take?'

As you try to foster participation there are three points you should keep in mind:

First, there are some health education methods that are useful for encouraging participation. Meetings and group discussions are examples (see Chapter 5). These may be formal meetings called by village leaders. They may be informal friendly discussions with individuals and small groups. Visit people in their homes. Go to places where people gather to relax. Talk with them and listen. In this way you will learn about their problems. At meetings, encourage all views to be presented. Quiet people have just as good ideas as people who talk a lot. Whenever possible try to get everybody to agree (this is called 'consensus'), so that the final plan is acceptable to all. This too will help guarantee participation and commitment.

Second, when fostering participation, remember the local culture. The method of participation will depend on the culture. Take meetings, for example: in some cultures it is not acceptable for young people to voice their opinions in public. If this is the case, then you will need, through discussion with the people concerned, to find some other way in which young people may express themselves. Maybe the youth leader could speak privately with some of the elders. You may also need to educate community leaders politely on the value of participation. Solving a problem is not easy and it may take a long time, but participation by the people will help a lot. Other examples of participation will be found in Chapters 3 and 6.

Finally, within communities it is important to encourage local leaders to play their part. If the problem affects the whole community, make sure that the planning group concerned is representative of all sections of it. Ways of identifying opinion leaders are discussed on pages 175–176. These people should lead the group in determining what are the main problems, then in developing solutions and plans to work them out. There should be a job for every member of the group. In this way no-one will feel left out. Everyone will then be committed to solving the problem. This will help more people gain skills and learn leadership responsibilities for the future. Follow-up is needed to check that each person has understood his or her job and does it well.

Action does not happen by itself. You will often need to encourage people to take responsibility.

Participation in evaluation

During a programme or planned activity, progress should be evaluated all the time. Similarly, at the end of a programme, success or failure must be measured (see pages 82–83, on how to do this). Participation plays its part here too. By discussing results with people, you can help them learn. If they know why a programme or action succeeded or failed, they will be able to make better efforts next time.

How much participation in health activities is there in your community now? How many people helped with the last big project? Do many people take responsibility, or do only a few do all the work? If participation is poor, why is this? What can you do to improve participation in your community? How best can the community health worker help promote participation?

Avoiding prejudice and bias

All people have prejudices. This problem was discussed briefly in Chapter 1. Prejudice means judging a person in advance simply because they are a member of a certain group. Prejudices are strong feelings either in favour of or against a person because of their age-group, tribe, religion, level of education, or place of birth. To succeed with health education, you must be aware of your own prejudices and attitudes. It may be difficult, but you should not let them influence you in your work. You should not favour one group above another. Above all, do not let your prejudices bring pain or damage to the communities you are trying to serve. Here is an example of what can happen if we let prejudices get in the way of our work.

Mrs Selma has been a health worker in the district for many years. One day she learns that there is a new community development worker in the district. The previous community development worker was a good friend to Mrs Selma. She was sorry to see her leave. The new community worker is very young. He has just finished training. Mrs Selma thinks to herself 'How can this young boy help our district? He is younger than my own son. I doubt if he will be very useful.'

Mrs Selma goes to the preschool clinic every day to talk with the mothers. On one particular day they were complaining that they needed skills so that they could earn more money to feed their children. Mrs Selma's first thought was of the community development workers. Her old friend always used to help over matters like this. But now she fears that the new community development worker will be too young and inexperienced to be of much help. She does not ask him to help.

Mrs Selma has a prejudice against the new community development worker. Because of her prejudice, she is probably hurting the mothers she wants to help. The community development worker is a valuable resource, but now the mothers will not be able to benefit from his help.

Here is another example.

Mr Tess is a health worker in a district where there are many villages. He is supposed to visit each village once a fortnight. He has many friends in Bola Village. He visits Bola once or twice a week. Because he visits Bola Village so often, he does not have time to visit some of the other villages. Mr Tess has a prejudice in favour of Bola Village. This prejudice causes him to neglect the needs of the other villages.

The third example shows that we should never let our biases bring gain to us, while bringing cost or pain to the community.

Mr Sam works in a local dispensary. He knows all the drugs very well. He is grateful to his uncle who helped him to go to school to learn his job. The uncle still gives him money sometimes. The uncle has a small drug store in the town. If patients come to the dispensary and the drugs they need are in short supply, Mr Sam will sometimes tell them to go to town to buy the drug in his uncle's store rather than try to get the drug for them. This will cost the patients more money.

Although Mr Sam has good reason to like his uncle, this is not a reason for allowing his bias to hurt the patients who come to him for help.

We must be careful about our prejudices and biases. They may affect the trust and relationship we have with the community. They may make our work in health education much more difficult. If we want everyone to participate in solving community health problems, we cannot let our prejudices and biases dominate our reason.

Through health education we should learn about our own behaviour too. We should try to improve ourselves so that we will be better able to serve the people and communities that need us.

Think about Mrs Selma, Mr Tess, and Mr Sam. What are the reasons for their prejudices and biases? Do you think that they can change their behaviour? It may be difficult. What would you recommend that each of them do so that their prejudices or biases will not harm the community? Is there someone else who could help?

What are your own prejudices—about other community health or social workers, about certain villages or neighbourhoods, about certain community leaders, about certain groups of people (young people, elders, people of the opposite sex, people from other areas, people of different religions)? Do you feel biased in favour of some people?

What can you do to make sure that your own prejudices or biases do not harm the people you are supposed to help?

Chapter 3

Planning for health education in primary health care

In health education we aim to encourage people to develop the confidence and skills to help themselves. In other words, the planning skills that are discussed in this chapter are not only for the use of health workers but also for the use of the community itself. Involving the community in the planning process is itself educational because once the skills have been learned and practised, the community will be able to take more initiative in planning its own programmes and activities. That is how self-reliance develops.

In this chapter eight basic planning skills are described:

● Collecting information (pages 40–53).

● Understanding problems (pages 54–58).

● Deciding on priorities, objectives, and action (pages 58–64).

● Identifying and obtaining resources (pages 64–71).

● Encouraging action and follow-through (pages 71–74).

● Selecting appropriate methods (pages 74–80).

● Evaluating results (pages 80–83).

● Reviewing the process of planning (pages 83–86).

These skills should not be seen as steps to be followed in a 1, 2, 3 order. Of course information must be collected before action can begin, but evaluation, although listed near the end, should start at the beginning of the process so that progress or drawbacks can be charted all along.

The importance of using appropriate technology, the need for community involvement, the value of partnership between the community and the health worker, and the need to coordinate different levels of health planning are emphasized.

Collecting information

Good health education is based on facts. It would not be correct to say 'I feel that poor nutrition is a problem because so many mothers do not know which foods are good for their children.' There must be facts. How many children are poorly nourished? What do we mean by poorly nourished? How do you measure or check whether children are poorly nourished? How many mothers know what to feed their children? How many do not? If many children are poorly nourished, is lack of knowledge the only reason? You need this information at the beginning of a programme so that by the end you can easily measure any change and improvement.

What information do we need?

We need to find out what are:

- The most important problems as seen by the person, group, or community you are helping.

- Other problems that you yourself may see.

- Problems that other community workers see.

- The number of people who have these problems.

- The practices that may have led to the problems.

- Possible reasons for these practices.

- Other causes of the problems.

To find this information, you will need to learn all about the community where you work. Among other things you will want to know:

- Local beliefs and values that affect health.

- The kinds of behaviour that are acceptable in the local culture.

- Important local people and reasons for their importance.

- How decisions are made about local problems.

- Available health care services, both traditional and modern.

- Location of services.

- The main occupations for both men and women, the level of education in the community, and the quality of the housing, as these factors may help you learn something about the economic conditions of the people.

- Existing clubs, societies, and organizations.

- The religions practised locally.

- Local ways of sharing ideas and feelings.

Do you know all these things about the community where you work? How did you learn them? If you do not know them all, work together with other health and community workers to collect the information. Each person can be responsible for collecting different types of information about the community. After collecting the information, meet with people and discuss it. See what new things you have learned about the community where you work.

The importance of collecting information

A family would not decide to build a new house without first investigating the availability of land and the cost of materials. A doctor would not begin to treat a patient without first investigating the nature of the illness through such methods as observation, questioning, and laboratory tests. Similarly, health workers practising health education must also investigate a problem before starting a programme or activities to deal with it. Here are some of the reasons why.

- It is necessary to know how big the problem is (how many people are affected) and how serious or dangerous it is (how much death and damage are being caused). Clear information about the nature of a problem will make it easier to choose priorities.

- If information is collected about the nature and extent of the problem both before and after a programme, it will be possible to show what impact the programme has made.

• Information about the community will make it possible to choose the most appropriate way to deal with the problem ('strategy'), both as regards the problem itself and the culture in which the problem exists. You will find more about priorities and strategy on page 58.

How to collect information

There are three main ways of collecting information about people, groups, and communities. First, there is observation, which is the collection of information by watching and listening. Secondly, there is interviewing, which involves discussion and questioning. Thirdly, there are records and documents, which are the written observations and experiences of other people.

These three methods are often used together in order to give a complete picture of a problem or survey of a community and its needs. For example regarding the problem of waterborne diseases, it would be useful to interview people about where they collect their water and how they store it. Secondly, it would be valuable to observe the various local sources of water to see if, in fact, people use them in the way they said they used them in the interview. Finally, records at the clinic would give an idea of the number of people actually suffering from waterborne diseases.

Observation

Know what and how to observe
Observation must be done carefully. Decide in advance what to observe, and how it will be observed. For example, parents and teachers may complain that children are passing blood in their urine. This may be caused by schistosomiasis, a disease caught by wading in streams (or ponds) contaminated by people infected by the disease defecating or urinating into the water. In this case it would be important (i) to observe whether the snails that harbour the disease are to be found in the streams, and (ii) to watch the behaviour of the children around the streams. If observation shows that there are disease-carrying snails and that children do play and wade in the streams and defecate or urinate in or near them, then one can rightly suspect schistosomiasis. Another form of observation would be to look at samples of urine or faeces under the microscope.

The local market should be included in any community survey, many health problems can be identified, and important information can be gathered. For example from a study of the market you can find out what food is available locally, and at what price, and you may be able to identify hazards that cause disease.

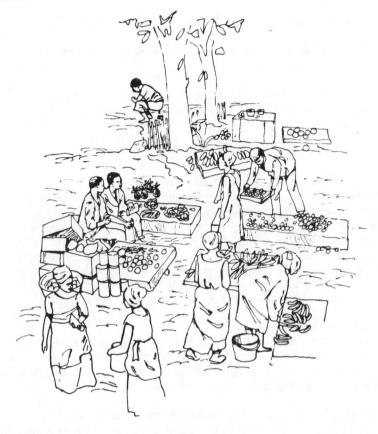

The local market should be included in any community survey. Many potential health hazards can be identified. What problems can you observe in this picture?.

Know when to observe

Observing at the wrong time may give the wrong impression about a problem. Observing a stream during school hours will not give a clear picture of children's wading and swimming behaviour. The best time to observe would be after school and at weekends when children are free to go to a stream if they wish.

Observe thoroughly and accurately

As pointed out above, observation is not only through the eyes. Important information can also be picked up through the ears, nose, fingers and tongue. Sound, smell, feeling and taste will teach you many things about your community. You should be able to tell people accurately what you have observed. For example, a health inspector sent three sanitary workers to look at a family's house. This is what each said:

- The first person reported 'the area was very dirty'.

- The second said 'the house was no worse than any others in the neighbourhood'.

- The third person said 'the gutter in front of the house was full of leaves and paper. Behind the house was a pile of tins, broken bottles, paper and rags that was as high as my knee and as wide as I am tall. All the rubbish was in this pile. None was scattered around the house.'

The three men observed the same thing, but their comments were different. The first two men made judgements. They did not report their observations completely. Only the third man gave a fairly accurate description. After you have observed something, think carefully about what you have seen; you may even want to write down your observations. Then decide whether what you saw was good or bad. Ask other people to observe the same thing and see if you all agree on what you saw or heard. Having others check your observations helps improve accuracy.

Observe individuals
Observation is very useful when you are helping individuals who are sick or have problems. The movements of their eyes and body can tell you much. Through observation you can see the signs of sadness, joy, worry, pain, fear, and other feelings.

Through observation you may also learn about a person's personal hygiene or attitude to health problems. For example, by observing cuts and wounds, you can tell if they are fresh, or if the person delayed coming to you. You can sometimes see whether traditional medicine has been used. Some people wear certain charms or symbols that tell you something about their beliefs and religion.

Sometimes you can learn about a person's financial condition or ethnic background by observing the style and condition of the clothes he or she is wearing. But be careful: if your eyes can teach you, they can also mislead you. Remember we all have prejudices. Clothing alone is not a sign of wealth or poverty, for example. Ask questions to see if your judgements are correct.

Observe groups
Use your eyes when you work with groups or committees. You can see whether some people are paying attention. Use your ears

to hear if people are participating. You can observe whether the group is happy or angry. If you observe problems you can then help to solve them.

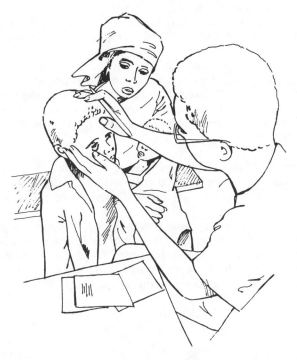

Observation of individual patients is important. Use your eyes to learn how the patient feels and see what modern or traditional remedies may have been tried.

It is useful to practise your observation skills. Gather a couple of friends or co-workers together. Choose one street in your village or neighbourhood. All of you walk along the street and observe it from the standpoint of environmental sanitation. Do not speak to each other until you reach the end of the street. Then discuss what you have observed. See if you have observed the same things. Walk back down the street to check your observations.

Use your eyes. Do you see scraps of paper or old tins lying about? Do you see blocked drains?

Use your nose. Do you smell garbage, stagnant water, or human wastes?

Use your ears. Do you hear many flies buzzing or goats, sheep, or dogs rummaging around in waste?

Involving other people in observation

Observation provides a good opportunity for participation and learning. Patients attending clinics can be encouraged to observe their own home environments. Community groups can be mobilized to observe their surroundings and undertake a community survey in order to discover problems and needs.

If the members of the community participate in collecting information, they will learn more about the problems facing their community. They will discover resources that meet their needs. They will gain ideas from community members about how to solve problems. And they will feel really involved in planning health activities.

The very best thing is when the people themselves start the survey, discuss their needs, determine with the health workers which needs are the most urgent, and then make plans.

A survey can be done by one person, but it takes a long time. It is best to have a small group. A school club could survey the community to learn what club-members could do to improve their village or neighbourhood. Community leaders themselves could also participate in conducting a survey.

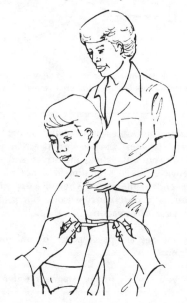

Participation should be encouraged when you are collecting information in a community about health and other needs. Schoolchildren, for instance, can be trained to use arm circumference bands. They could then participate in finding out how well or poorly nourished the pre-school children in the community are.

It is not enough simply to collect information. The information must be studied carefully so that people can learn from it. Hold discussions with the people. Share ideas. Help people reach some conclusions about what problems are most serious and why those problems exist. Find out if their survey has suggested any resources that could be used in solving the problems.

Interviewing people

An interview is a way of gathering information through communication between someone who wants information (the interviewer) and people who can supply the information (the interviewees).

Your relationship skills are most important for interviewing. If a person does not trust you, he or she may not talk freely and may give false information. Always make sure the person knows who you are and why you want to talk to him or her.

An interview must be planned carefully. Interviewing may involve talking to a group of people at the market or a special meeting with a village leader over a serious community problem. In either case you must have a clear idea beforehand about what information you are trying to obtain.

What to ask

You will probably find that you need two types of information. At the beginning of a programme it is likely that you will be seeking general information. This may concern the way of life in the community and the various needs that people see.

Later you may be seeking specific information. Through general interviewing you may have found, for example, that many people feel that the town needs a new market. A specific interview would aim at finding out what problems there are with the present market; the action that has already been taken; ideas for improving the market; and the contributions that people are willing to make to solving the problems.

Who to interview

Next you must decide who to interview. People can be interviewed in groups. If the concern is a new market, you could attend a meeting of the association of people who sell at the market, and ask them if they would discuss their ideas and feelings with you. If they agree, you can go ahead with an interview in which you will collect information more quickly than if you had had to talk to individuals.

A group interview can be a starting-point for solving community problems. Not only can group members identify pressing problems. They can also discuss and come to understand the reasons why these problems exist. Once this is done, the group can go on to discuss possible solutions.

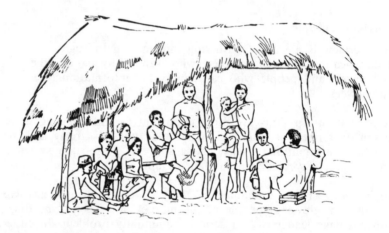

Interviewing a group of people at a community meeting is one way of gathering information about community needs and problems. Here, the residents of a village have gathered to share their concerns with a community health worker.

At other times an individual interview is necessary. Not everyone will be willing to share their true opinions in a group. In our market example, views may be very diverse and talking in a group may cause a lot of anger. In such a case, it would be better to find out through individual interviews what each person really wants. An individual interview is of course the usual way of helping patients who come to you for health care.

In addition to interviewing the general population, it is very important to interview local leaders. Also talk to people who have accepted new ideas such as family planning methods or ventilated latrines. Find out why they accepted these new ideas. This will help you learn about the process of change in your community.

If you are seeking the ideas of many people concerning a problem, set out the topics you want to discuss and the questions you want to ask, before going to meet them. Then be sure to ask the same questions in the same way to each person. Questions asked in different ways to different people will result in many different and confusing answers. If that happens, the information will be useless.

How to ask for information

Interviewing uses questions and comments to encourage people to supply information. The words used must be chosen carefully, because words influence how a person answers.

There are four types of question or comment, but not all of these will yield useful information.

Let us take once again the example of the market to see how these four types of question could be used to gain specific information about the problem. As you will see, some approaches are better than others.

'Does our village need a new market?'

This is a *simple direct question* that could be answered with a simple 'Yes' or 'No'. But starting an interview with this type of question may bring problems. First, people may try to guess the opinion of the interviewer or the village leaders and answer in the way they think they are supposed to, not the way they really feel.

Secondly, this type of question does not give room for discussion. An answer of 'Yes' or 'No', does not show the full range of feelings and opinions a person has on the subject. A person may answer 'yes', but in fact feel that the market is not the most important problem in the village at that moment. A direct question will not encourage the expression of that opinion.

It is best to save direct questions for later on in the interview. After the person has begun sharing opinions freely, a direct question can then be used to help clarify points.

'Don't you feel our village needs a new market?'

This is a *leading question* because it leads a person to give only one answer. People easily say "Yes" to such a question. Questions that start like this:

'Don't you think . . .', 'Isn't it true . . .', 'Wouldn't you believe . . .', 'Shouldn't you have . . .': make people give one-sided answers. They are dangerous to use in interviews because interviewees will almost always agree and rarely reveal their true opinion.

'Should our village have a new market this year or next year?'

This is a *forced-choice question*. It gives the interviewee a choice of only two answers – 'this year' or 'next year'. People being

49

interviewed will almost certainly make one of the choices, although they may have a completely different opinion. They may really want to say 'in five years' or even 'never'.

'Please tell me your views about our market.'

This is an approach that leads to *open comments*. Such a statement allows people to answer freely. Listen carefully so that people will be encouraged to express their views fully.

After a person has expressed some ideas, you might say, 'That is interesting. Could you tell me more?' You might also use *direct questions* now that the person has felt free to talk.

Suppose you were interviewing a mother about her sick child. You observe that the child is quite small for its age, so you want to find out more about what the child is eating. Opposite are some sample questions and statements that might start off an interview with the mother. Put an X in the column you consider appropriate; questions that should never be used; questions that may be used at the beginning of the interview; and those that may be used later in the interview.

Think carefully about the reasons why you marked the statements the way you did. Discuss this among your co-workers. Then compare your list with the answers below.

Now assume that you will be interviewing a member of the local farmers' cooperative. The farmers have been having problems with snakebites. Make up some sample questions and comments that you could use to start the interview.

You could also have a role-play on the subject with a friend or co-worker pretending to be the farmer you are interviewing (see page 152 for details on role-playing). Get others to watch you. They can tell you if your comments and questions were good, or whether they made the other person give one-sided or false answers.

> Here are the answers to the statements and questions on page 51. You should have put 'X' in the first column for these numbers: 4, 6, 7, 11, 12; in the second column for 2, 5, 8, 10; and in the third column for 1, 3, 9 (5 could go here also).

Sample questions and statements	When would you use the questions and statements?		
	Never	To start with	Later
1. Does the baby eat fruit?			
2. Welcome to the clinic.			
3. How many times a day does the baby eat?			
4. Don't you give the child eggs?			
5. Please tell me about the child's favourite foods.			
6. Do you give cereal, eggs, or bread for breakfast?			
7. Shouldn't this child be eating more beans?			
8. Let us discuss your child's feeding habits so both of us can learn how best to keep him healthy.			
9. Are there any foods the child refuses?			
10. Please tell me about any problems you may have in feeding this child.			
11. Does the child eat most in the morning or afternoon?			
12. Wouldn't it be better if this child could eat more meat?			

Using records and documents

Written information can help us learn much about the people and communities with whom we are working. Most agencies and organizations keep records and reports of their activities. By looking through these, we can sometimes discover something about the nature of health problems. For example, we may see that certain diseases are more prevalent at certain times of the year, giving us ideas on when to plan action.

Some examples of records are: files on patients at the clinic; annual reports of agencies; monthly figures on clinic attendance and common diseases; newspaper reports on important events; written programme plans; agency reports on the use of drugs and supplies; absentee reports from schools and work-places; and certain books, pamphlets, and magazines.

Useful records for working with individuals

You may be working in a health centre. A mother brings in a child who has diarrhoea (frequent watery stools). The child's card may give information that would help in understanding and solving the problem. Check how many times the child has had diarrhoea. If the child has come to the health centre several times in the past year with the same complaint, then it might be reasonable to suspect, among other things, that there is something wrong with the sanitation of the home. This clue could be followed up by an interview about hygienic practices in the home, and a home visit.

The child's recorded weight would be another useful piece of information. A sudden drop or no gain for several months should cause concern. Possible reasons for a drop may be: the child's illness; removal of the child from breast-feeding, with a poor weaning diet; a family financial crisis; or a death in the family. The weight record provides a clue to the problem which can then be followed up with an interview.

Medicaments prescribed at previous visits are also recorded on patients' cards. This information can be used to find out whether the patient has taken the drugs correctly, benefited from them, or suffered side-effects. Such information is useful for planning future treatment. Finally, look for other useful information such as personal and family history, plus the recorded observations of previous health workers.

Useful records for working with groups

School attendance records will show whether many children have been absent recently and from which classes. If absence is high or shows a change from the normal pattern, it should be investigated. The school curriculum is a document of what the Ministry of Education thinks children should be taught. Look at the curriculum and compare it, through observation and interview, with what is really being taught about health.

The records of a farmers' cooperative would give an idea of the farmers' needs. Food production is related to nutrition and health. Records of the types of food crop and the amount produced will show where improvements could be made.

Clinic records may also help you understand the problems and needs of a group of farmers. Look in these records for complaints common to farmers, such as hookworm and snakebite.

Useful records for determining community needs

At the community level, clinic records show the main diseases people are reporting. Study the records of past years to see if diseases have been increasing or decreasing. Remember, though, that not everyone attends the clinic. The records there may not tell you the whole story about a community's health problems.

Another source of information is offered by annual reports, pamphlets, and other material from government and voluntary agencies. These will tell you about the programmes that are organized to meet your community's problems.

Visit your local health centre or clinic. Find out what kind of records are kept and what kinds of reports are sent to the regional or state headquarters. Ask to see some of the reports and study them with the following questions in mind.

What are the most common health problems? Which cause the most illness? Which are the most serious and cause the most death and disability?

Are there clinic attendance figures? Is attendance increasing, decreasing, or staying the same? What might be the reasons?

Do you think the clinic records accurately show the community's health needs? Are there many people who do not go to the clinic when they are sick?

Do your community leaders know what are the most common and most serious problems seen at the clinic? If they don't, how can you help them learn about these problems?

Visit the local schools. What kinds of records do they have? What can you learn from those records?

Understanding problems

Unless you understand clearly what factors are involved in a problem, you will not be able to control it. There are different causes that must be examined.

Why are there problems?

The most important word in this section is why. Information collected about the community or about individuals will show that some things are going well but that there are also many problems. Simply knowing that things are going well or badly is not enough for planning a programme.

It is important to know why a community project, for example, is succeeding or why people are healthy, so that you can learn from such information and promote similar successes in the future. In the same way, one must know why there are problems so that the most appropriate steps can be taken to find solutions.

Chapter 1 was written to help understand why problems occur, and why they don't. Read the four examples below. Look back to Chapter 1 and see if you can think of some possible explanations why some of the people in the examples have problems while others do not.

In one village 50 out of 100 mothers bring their children for monthly appointments at the child welfare clinic. In another village, 85 out of 100 mothers attend. Why?

One man has come to the clinic complaining of roundworm twice in the past year. His neighbour has never had this problem. Why?

In October, there were very few people with a cough in one village. By March, there were three times as many people with a cough. Why?

In one village the people have built their own latrines, wells, and school. A nearby village has none of these things. Why?

Involving the community

It is not only the health or community worker who must understand why problems do or do not occur. The members of the community must also understand. Meetings and discussions with individuals, groups, or community representatives are useful for helping people look closely at the reasons for problems. In this way information gathered about the community can be shared and examined. When community members learn more about their problems, they will be better able to make good choices on action to solve them.

The role of behaviour

Like beliefs, some kinds of behaviour may promote health and some may lead to illness, while the effect of others may be neutral or at least unknown. We discussed this in Chapter 1.

When looking at health behaviour, the first thing is to understand why people take certain actions that promote health. What resources, beliefs, values, and important people encourage healthy behaviour or make it possible? What activities can be planned to support and strengthen healthy practices?

Next comes consideration of unhealthy behaviour. If people have shown that they want to improve the situation, at least three things could be done about unhealthy practices:

- Ignore the unhealthy behaviour, and encourage instead an existing alternative way of behaving that is healthy.

- Slightly change the unhealthy behaviour to remove some of its more dangerous aspects.

- Substitute completely new practices for the unhealthy ones.

An understanding of the situation is needed to help in deciding which of these actions would be the best. Since behaviour is part of the way of life or culture of a community, the best step may be to encourage already existing healthy practices as an alternative to unhealthy ones. If no appropriate or acceptable alternatives exist, the next choice would be to find ways of slightly changing the harmful behaviour. The most difficult line of action of the three is for people to try substituting completely new practices for old familiar ones.

Here is an example of how a good understanding of behaviour can lead to appropriate action.

In one village the traditional midwives always used pieces of green glass to cut the umbilical cord of newborns. They believed that the glass had certain magic powers that protected the baby. Unfortunately, this village also had a high incidence of neonatal tetanus.

During a discussion, the midwives admitted that they were worried about tetanus, but did not know what to do. Were any other methods of cutting the cord used?

No others were used in that village, but one woman mentioned that in nearby villages some midwives used knives. An elderly midwife then reminded the group that she believed that metal held evil spirits that could harm a young baby. Thus a knife was not an acceptable alternative. At this point the health worker who was attending the discussion realized that substituting a new practice such as the use of clean razor blades would not work, because they were made of metal. Possibly the existing practice could be slightly changed? The sharp pieces of broken glass certainly could cut the cord almost as well as a razor blade. The problem was that a dirty piece of glass could cause tetanus. A simple change could be to put the glass, before use, in boiling water for at least ten minutes to kill the tetanus spores. This was acceptable to the midwives.

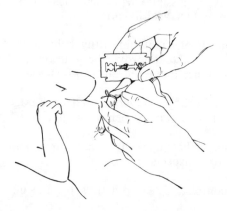

Using a clean, new razor blade to cut the umbilical cord of a newborn baby is a healthy practice which traditional midwives could adopt if local practices are not safe. It is often possible to modify traditional practices or find alternatives that would be equally safe and more in line with local beliefs and culture.

Who can solve problems?

Some problems can be solved by individual effort alone, while others require the assistance or cooperation of several people, or of the whole community. For example, a community may be experiencing the bad effects of poor environmental sanitation. The behaviour of individuals and families contributes to the problem because waste and faeces are spread about everywhere. In solving the problem, the whole community may need to set up a waste collection system and to provide latrine facilities through cooperative action. Then it would be the responsibility of individuals and families to make hygienic use of these facilities. Here are other examples:

- An individual can take responsibility for personal hygiene.

- Good nutrition is usually the responsibility of the whole family.

- In order to rent a tractor, a group of farmers may have to share the cost.

- Guaranteeing a safe water supply is the responsibility of the community.

- The national government, through the ministry of health, is responsible for providing vaccines.

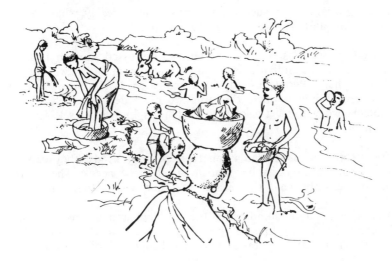

Sometimes the whole community may have to take action to solve a problem. This is the case when the problem is associated with unhealthy practices that are usual and accepted in the community.

What is the type of help needed?

Look at a disease like tuberculosis. Some people in the community may have recently fallen ill with the disease. They need treatment. They need to take their drugs regularly. They have lost weight, have become very weak, and may even have lost their jobs. They need rehabilitation to help them recover their health and jobs so that they may live a normal life again. Many are not sick, but they need to take preventive action to keep well. This includes not only immunization, but also health promotion measures such as adequate nutrition.

You can see that different kinds of behaviour are needed depending on whether we want to prevent tuberculosis, treat the disease, or provide rehabilitation. This is true for most problems.

Try to understand the appropriate behaviour at each stage of the problem. Plan education programmes to help people adopt the kind of behaviour that will prevent them from becoming ill, cure them if they are sick, and help them lead normal lives if they are disabled.

Deciding on priorities, objectives, and action

For a programme to succeed, we must know clearly what we want to do and how we are going to do it.

In the first sections of this chapter, we discussed how to find out the needs of the individuals, groups, and communities we are trying to help. People usually have many needs. It is not possible to do everything at once, therefore we must decide which problems we will try to solve first. This is known as setting priorities.

After people have decided upon their priority needs, they can think about what must be done to meet those needs. They must spell out exactly what they want – in other words, their objectives.

Then with an understanding of the problem and an eye on the objectives, they can consider how best to deal with the problem, that is, what action to take. This is called developing a strategy.

People must determine what their priorities and objectives are, and what strategies are acceptable to them. To do this, they need professional help, but the members of the community must make the final choices.

Setting priorities

Setting priorities with individuals

It is not always easy to know what problem to face first. People have many pressing problems like those of the family described opposite.

Mrs Antia has five children. The oldest is eight years old, and the youngest nine months. Mrs Antia is pregnant again. The family shares one room, made of boards and metal roofing-sheets, stuck on the back of the house of Mr Antia's father. Mrs Antia is not very strong these days. She has not had a regular job for the past four years.

Mr Antia is a fisherman. He has not been very successful with his fishing lately. Now he spends several months at a time working in the city as a daily paid labourer. The small amount of money he brings back from the city is hardly enough to feed the family. In fact the children are all underweight and sickly.

Mr and Mrs Antia discuss their problems with a health worker. These are some of the needs they mention:

- A bigger place to live in.
- More money.
- A job for Mrs Antia.
- Skills for Mr Antia so that he can get a better job.
- Food for the children.
- Medicine for the children.
- Medicine and rest for Mrs Antia.
- A way to stop the family growing in size.
- New clothing so that other villagers will respect the family.
- A radio for Mrs Antia, to relieve her loneliness.

At first some of these needs clearly seem more important than others, but priorities cannot be chosen only on what seems or feels right. There must be a reason for the choice. Below are four questions that can help people see their problems more clearly and make their choice of priorities easier. Note that during discussion people will come to realize that many of their needs are related. Satisfying a priority need may in fact solve many other problems as well.

Which is the most serious problem?
For the Antia family, lack of food may be the most serious problem. Poorly fed children will be susceptible to many diseases which may handicap them for the rest of their lives.

Where does the greatest future benefit lie?
Concern is not only for temporarily solving problems today, but for making the future brighter. Providing Mr Antia with skills so that he could get a better-paid job would give benefit now and in the future.

What needs can be met with the resources available?
The Antia family has little money, and Mrs Antia is unlikely to get a job now. With their existing resources they probably cannot afford new clothes and a radio. They cannot even afford certain foods. But, within their resources, there are inexpensive, yet nutritious foods available at the local market.

59

Which are the problems of greatest concern to the people?
Mrs Antia is most interested in the radio, but both she and her husband are interested in getting a better-paid job for Mr Antia. People are more likely to take action to solve problems in which they have an interest than those in which they do not. Also the more people there are who take interest, the more likely it is that the problem can be solved.

After considering all these questions together, Mr and Mrs Antia decided that job training for Mr Antia and buying more nutritious foods within their present budget were their immediate priorities.

Setting priorities with communities

The same four questions should be considered at meetings in which communities are discussing their priorities. When more people are involved, there will be more views to consider. It may take longer to decide on priorities than when only one or two people are concerned.

Educational games can help make clear what is involved in setting community priorities. Such games can be played with a group of health and community workers, with a class of high school students, or even with a group of community leaders. An example is given below of their specific use in helping communities to select priorities, objectives, and strategies.

A simple scenario can be developed from a case study of a small village with many problems. Everyone who plays the game takes the role of a village member. Each person chooses a different occupation and identity and is asked to express his or her own opinion about which are the most important needs, and why, and what is a priority for immediate action. As the game progresses, it will become evident that people with different backgrounds and opinions will see more benefit in one problem being solved than in another. This will make the discussion lively. Around twenty is a good number for playing this game. Of course you can create as many parts as you need, depending on the number of people in the group.

First, slowly read to the group the story of the village (see page 61). Assign each person a role such as farmer, barber, weaver, or food-seller. Then read the story aloud again, and read the four questions listed on pages 59–60. Ask everyone to think about them. The group should then have a discussion and try to agree on one or two top priorities. People do not have to sit in a large group. They may break into small interest groups. Some may move back and forth between groups trying to get support for their own ideas. You should move around and listen. Remind people about the four questions on choosing priorities (you might write them on a board or poster, if people can read). Also remind people that meeting needs usually costs time and money. Encourage players to find the least expensive ways of meeting the needs with the resources available.

Allow the game to go on for about an hour. After that time, stop the discussion even if no priorities have been chosen. Discuss with the participants what they have learned about setting priorities. Discuss how the group could improve its priority-setting skills.

Here is the story of Poro Village which you can use as it is or adapt to make the village sound more like those in the area where you are working.

> Poro is a small rural village of 300 people. It has a big market which used to attract people from all over the surrounding area. Unfortunately the five kilometres of dirt road leading into Poro have become very rough. Fewer people are coming now, so business at the market is not good and the villagers are losing money. The road needs repairing.
>
> The closest water source is a stream two kilometres away which dries up at certain times of year. The main town of the district, about ten kilometres away, has a piped water supply. The residents of Poro feel that they deserve the same.
>
> The nearest school to Poro is in another village reached by a path through the forest. Children using the path have been bitten by snakes and injured through tripping over fallen trees. People in Poro want their own school.
>
> The nearest health centre is in the main town. This is far to travel for a sick person, and the health workers who promise to visit Poro never come. The villagers want a health centre too.
>
> Finally, because the main town of the district has electricity, people feel that Poro should have electricity too. This would help their children study and make life at night more interesting.

Here are some of the roles people can play: farmer, carpenter, baker, weaver, potter, tailor, trader, seamstress, food seller, religious leader, chief (or political leader), bicycle repairer, mason, herbalist, shopkeeper, midwife, housewife.

Setting objectives

If at the beginning of a programme people have a clear idea of what they want, by the end of the programme they will know if they have succeeded. An objective is exactly what people want to see achieved by the end of the programme.

Health objectives

The result of a primary health care programme should be an improvement in the people's health. For example, if measles is a serious problem in a community, a programme to solve the problem might have the following as its health objectives:

- Fewer children will get measles.

- Those who do get measles will recover quickly and suffer no disabilities.

- No children will die from measles.

Educational objectives

Since people's behaviour affects their health, there will be certain actions that people must carry out to solve their health problems.

Such actions are the educational objectives of a programme. Here are some examples of educational objectives for a programme against measles:

- Mothers will bring their children for immunization.

- Mothers whose children get measles will bring them quickly to the health worker for care.

- To prevent blindness, mothers will keep children who have measles in a darkened room and make sure that they rest.

- Children who get measles will be fed as well as possible to help them recover more quickly.

Participation in setting objectives

The individuals, groups, or communities with whom you are working should be encouraged to select their own objectives and receive guidance on doing so. This is only reasonable, since they are the ones who are experiencing a problem.

When people set their own objectives, it is more likely that the health behaviour they decide upon will fit with the local culture and available resources. As a guide, the role of the health worker is always to encourage people to examine and discuss the feasibility of the objectives, in other words whether the objectives chosen are likely to be achieved.

It may be some months before the results of activities can be seen. Remind people of this so that they are not disappointed if things haven't changed as soon as the initial action is finished.

Some factors in success

Looking at existing alternative practices is one way of ensuring a successful outcome. Supposing that a group of mothers want their children to grow bigger and healthier. As part of a balanced diet they would need to include enough protein foods. There are many alternative forms of protein that they can include in the normal diet: beans, meat, groundnuts, milk, seeds, cheese, chicken, fish, snails, and certain insects.

A health worker could guide the mothers in their choice by asking questions like: At what times of the year are these different foods available? What is the price of these foods? Is it against local beliefs for children to eat any of these foods? Can these foods be easily prepared by the mothers? Which of the foods do children actually like? Through such a discussion, feasible objectives could be set regarding exactly what foods mothers should try to give their children.

You have probably realized that, for the mothers to achieve their objectives, other people must also act. Perhaps fathers will have to provide money. Perhaps mothers-in-law will have to be convinced. Farmers are also involved: the ministry of agriculture may have to provide loans and expert advice to local farmers producing the food. The Ministry of Labour or Social Development may have to help mothers and fathers find better ways to earn money so that they can buy food. Objectives need to be set at the individual, community, and national level, because all must play their part.

The steps to take to achieve objectives

Decisions on what steps to take—that is on the most appropriate 'strategy'—will be based on the different reasons behind behaviour that causes health problems. It will also take other factors into consideration, such as the local culture, economic problems, etc.

The chart below explains this idea. It includes suggestions for educational methods, that will be discussed in detail in Chapter 7. Some of the methods are also discussed briefly in this chapter and in Chapters 5 and 6.

Since problems often have several causes, it may be necessary to use different strategies in a programme. Also note that although certain educational methods are listed next to certain types of action, they can also be used with others. However, some methods work better with one type of problem than with another.

Problem	Type of action needed (strategy)	Possible educational methods
Lack of knowledge	Information	Posters, radio, press, talks, displays
Influence of other people	Support	Discussion groups, clubs, family counselling
Lack of skills	Training	Demonstrations, case studies, educational games
Lack of resources	Development	Community surveys, community meeting, resource-linking
Conflict with values	Clarification of values	Role-playing, educational games, stories

Identifying and obtaining resources

In the first chapter we discussed the important effect that the presence or absence of resources can have on behaviour. This section looks at ways of finding the resources necessary to promote health, and conduct health education programmes.

Resources inside the community

Be aware of the resources within your own community that can be used in solving the problems of individuals, of groups, or of the whole village.

Here are some examples of the many kinds of resources you will need:

● Places to hold meetings, discussions, and training sessions, such as schools, and town halls.

● Some people may be able to donate money to buy materials.

- Some people may have skills that would be useful for community projects. Among these are carpenters, teachers, masons, artists, traditional healers, weavers, and potters.

- Many able-bodied people can give their labour.

- Some people may own bicycles, motor cycles, or other vehicles. Transport is valuable for carrying materials for projects or taking sick people to the clinic.

- Materials such as wood, cloth, and food can be given by people for large community projects, or to help families in times of crisis; for treating sick people you may find that some local herbs work very well; you can encourage people to make tools and equipment for their projects.

Make sure you know who has any of these resources, and how they can be obtained. As can be seen from the list above, the members of the community themselves are the most important resources for solving problems.

Resources outside the community

It is best to solve problems with resources from within your own community. Sometimes, though, the project may be too big for the resources available. Also the problem may be difficult to solve. Then it is necessary to look outside. Here are some resources you may find outside your community:

- Some agencies and ministries give funds and technical assistance for community projects or for individuals and families in need.

- People with skills, such as finding underground water for wells, may come from outside.

- Materials such as cement may have to come from outside as well; for educational material such as films and posters, you may look to different agencies; vaccines, drugs, and medical equipment are sent from outside; many kinds of machines and equipment are sold, loaned, or given by outside agencies.

Appropriate resources

We have said that it is best to find resources inside your community. For one thing, it saves money. But, more important yet, people are proud to be able to help themselves. This pride

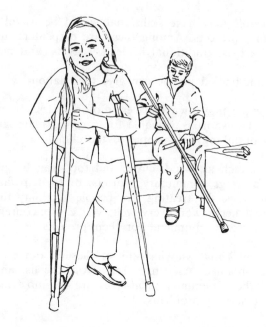

Use local resources to solve problems. Carpenters in this community have helped by making crutches for handicapped children.

will encourage people to try to solve more problems by their own efforts.

It may not be necessary to buy cement outside to make incinerators, for example. Mud, clay, bricks, and stone are appropriate local building materials.

A tractor may look like a wonderful answer to farmers' problems. After some time though, they may be disappointed when they see the cost of petrol and the difficulty of getting repairs when the tractor breaks down. An improved design for local ploughs or the use of horses, mules, oxen, or buffalos might be more appropriate and have better long-term results.

Linking people with resources

Once resources have been found that will help solve the problem of the person, the group, or the community in need, you must still bring the people and the resources together. Good relationships with people and communication skills are very important here. Only through good relations can you bring together the people in need with the people who have the resources.

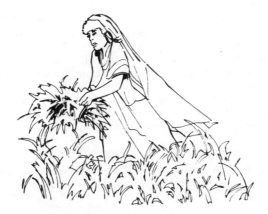

This woman is collecting special leaves and grasses that can be used to make medicine. These are often a valuable local resource.

When we talked about participation, we said that it was a mistake to do work for people that they can do for themselves. This is true with resources, too. Do not get resources for people if they can get them for themselves. If you do it for them, they may not be able to find help the next time they are in need. This is what happened to one community worker, Mr Neb.

Mr Neb was talking one day to a farmers' cooperative in his district. The farmers said that they needed money to buy seeds and fertilizers. Mr Neb promised he would help. He went to the Ministry of Agriculture and found the section that gives loans to farmers. He got the forms and brought them back. After asking the farmers a few questions, he filled in the forms for them. He took the forms back to the ministry and got the money for the farmers.

Later that year Mr Neb was transferred to another district. When the time came to repay the loan, the farmers did not know what to do. Only Mr Neb knew all about the resources at the ministry. Finally, an angry official from the ministry came to collect the money. The farmers gave it to him, but were afraid to ask him more about loans because they could see his anger. When the next planting season came, the farmers did not know how to get a loan.

Sometimes problems become more confused when a health worker tries to get people a resource that they could have obtained themselves. This is what happened to Mrs Sandos.

Mrs Sandos, a community midwife, heard that people in her community needed a reliable well. She volunteered to go to the provincial capital to seek help at the Ministry of Public Works. An official at the ministry gave Mrs Sandos plans for a well. The officer also promised to help with costs and supplies if the villagers dug the well exactly to plan.

The villagers were happy to receive Mrs Sandos' report and began digging the well right away. Before they were half-way down to the depth required by the plan, they struck water. Though they tried, they could not go deeper. When Mrs Sandos reported back to the ministry, the official said that he would not give any help now, because the well was not dug according to the plans. Mrs Sandos tried to explain the problem, but the officer would not listen. Mrs Sandos was embarassed to return home with the bad news and, when she did, the villagers accused her of lying. They gave up interest in the project and today they still have no reliable well.

> Think about these two stories. What could the two health workers have done to make a better link between village and resource?

Actually there are several things that you can do to assist individuals, groups, and whole communities in learning to link up with resources. First you must supply background information that will help people to make an effective link. Such information should include:

- Names of agencies, organizations, and individuals that have resources.

- Description of type of resources provided.

- Location of the resource agency.

- Special requirements the agency may have before giving resources.

Selecting the best resources

Discuss the benefits and difficulties that might come with each resource and what is best considering the culture and needs of the community itself. The people involved should make the decision. Do not force an idea on the people.

Exploratory visit

The community will learn more about the resource if a visit is made to the agency that has the resource. While you may provide some background information, it is better if the people learn at first hand what the resource agency offers.

You should not go to the resource agency alone. If the villagers are not confident enough to go by themselves, you can go with them the first time. But they must soon learn to go by themselves. If you are working with a group, the group may send

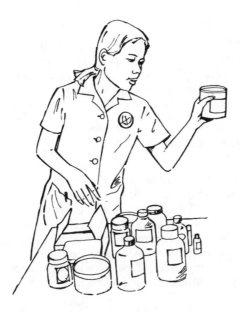

Many different resources can be used to solve a problem. For example this health worker has many drugs to choose from when supplying a community medicine kit. The pharmacist can help her choose the most appropriate ones for her community.

a few representatives to see the resource agency. You can introduce the people but should encourage them to speak for themselves. The person or the group who made the visit will report back and encourage further discussion.

Obtaining the resource

The people should make their own decision whether to accept the resource or not. They themselves should also make all arrangements directly with the agency. You can be with the people to make sure that they understand what is happening and that no-one is taking unfair advantage of them. People must know in advance what, if anything, the agency expects them to do in return.

Encouraging learning

At each step of the linking process, explain carefully to the people what is happening. Be sure that more than one person in a group or community knows how to link up with resources. Then, in case of sickness or travel, there will always be someone around who knows what to do.

Maintaining collaboration

Communities will benefit from the resources of many different agencies—education, agriculture, social development, information, public works, and a variety of voluntary and special purpose organizations. Help the community establish ongoing links with these different agencies.

Health education resources

In this section we have talked about resources needed to achieve actual programme goals—cement for a well, or volunteer labour to build a community meeting-hall, for example. We must also remember that special resources are needed to communicate the health message that will encourage people to undertake the programme in the first place. All the points we have raised about general programme resources (type, availability, and appropriateness) also apply to education and communication resources.

Local media

When collecting information about the community, you should look for local and traditional means of communication. These may include proverbs, stories, and fables which elders use to pass traditional values on to the young. Local leaders may use town criers or bell-ringers to announce coming events. Traditional songs or plays may communicate important ideas and values. Some people may own a print shop and be able to make posters to inform the public. There may also be a photographer in the neighbourhood.

Consider which of these and other communication media are available in your community. Use the ones that will best support your health education efforts. By using locally available means of communication you will be involving the community in the programme. Get their ideas on which traditional proverbs, songs, or stories will be most appropriate for conveying the health message. Involve local leaders so that they would be willing to use their town criers to announce important health events and rally the community to take part. Local artists, printers, and photographers can be involved in designing, and producing educational material.

Outside resources

Also identify communication resources outside the community. These may include mass media such as newspapers and radio. The ministries of health and of information may have films, posters, and vans with loudspeakers that can be borrowed for local health education programmes. Find out who in the community has access to newspapers, radios, and other information sources. These people can be encouraged to share the health information they obtain. A local school-teacher who subscribes to a newspaper can save articles that relate to health and use them to teach pupils and inform parents. A community member who owns a radio could invite neighbours to listen when health programmes are broadcast.

You, as a local health worker, should be aware of such newspaper articles and radio programmes so that you can encourage community members to read and listen, and benefit from the information provided. This involves resource-linking. Contact the radio or television station and obtain their programme schedule. When health programmes are broadcast, encourage community members to listen. You may even encourage them to gather as a group to listen, so that after the programme a discussion can be held to make sure that everyone has understood the ideas presented.

Get in touch with the ministries of health and of information. Find out what resources they have and on what conditions they loan materials such as films. Read Chapter 7 to learn more about different educational media and communication resources.

Encouraging action and follow-through

If you have been following the steps described so far, you should have a strong foundation for your health education work. You know the problems, the priorities, the objectives, the resources. Now, all of this must be put together into a specific plan of action that will show what will be done, by whom, and when. In other words you need to prepare a timetable.

Preparing a timetable

Suppose your community feels that its most important health problem is the lack of a convenient drinking-water supply. The timetable on page 73 is an example of how to set out the timing of tasks and responsibilities. One thing to remember when setting target dates for various tasks is to be realistic. It takes time for people to get organized and it takes time to find resources. People will be disappointed if they set a schedule that is too short for the actual completion of the assigned tasks. A timetable is also useful in checking whether the programme is progressing as scheduled.

A copy of the timetable can be put up in the town hall or in another place where people will see it.

The timetable reproduced opposite was set up for a community programme, to improve the water supply. You can adapt the timetable and activities to your own community projects.

A timetable may even be drawn up for an individual; this would be less complicated than one for a community. An example is the case of a mother whose child is underweight. Together with the mother, you could work out a timetable showing the foods that might be prepared for the child each day. This might look like a one-week menu. On the same timetable you would also note follow-up clinic appointments.

If the mother could not read, you would not be able to write out a timetable for her, but you would discuss the schedule to help her remember. Also she might have a child or relative who is able to read. A timetable could then be written that someone could read to her.

Assigning tasks

When a programme involves more than one person, it is important to make sure as many people participate as possible.

In the timetable there is a column headed 'people responsible'. We used general terms like 'leaders', 'volunteers', and 'local people'. In a real timetable you would list the names of the people who have agreed to take responsibility for one task or another.

For example, with the community water supply project: Who will be on the fund-raising committee? Who will get the cement? Who will find the shovels? Who will be the volunteer workers? Who will be in charge of the volunteers?

Follow-through action

This involves the steps listed below:

● Set a specific date on which to start your main action.

Sample timetable for the provision of a community water supply

Tasks	Completed by	People responsible
1. Community leaders discuss the problem of waterborne diseases	1st week	community health workers
2. Leaders trained on cause and prevention	3rd week	community health workers
3. Public information activities begin, using local media and home visits	4th week	leaders, community health workers, schoolteachers
4. All sick people report for treatment	5th week	leaders, community health workers, local people
5. People boil and filter their water	6th week	leaders (one for each town/village/section)
6. Funds raised for well construction	12th week	fund-raising committee, leaders
7. Voluntary labour recruited	12th week	leaders
8. Well sites selected	12th week	leaders and local people
9. Materials obtained	15th week	materials committee
10. Construction begins	15th week	volunteer labourers, community health workers
11. Maintenance committee selected for each well	15th week	leaders
12. Maintenance committee members trained in maintenance of wells	16th week	health worker
13. Wells completed	20th week	volunteer labourers
14. People use water only from wells; maintain wells hygienically	20th week onwards	leaders and local people

- Be sure each person knows his or her duties: Can each person tell you from memory what he or she must do and when he or she will do it?

- Keep in contact with people; provide encouragement; answer questions; help solve problems.

- Hold regular meetings to review progress: at these meetings each responsible person can report on what he or she has done; the group can then compare each report with the timetable and see if the work is progressing according to schedule.

- If there is some delay in the schedule the group should look into the problem immediately: Can it be corrected at once? What are the needs? More materials? More volunteers? More time? More funds?

Remember that it is better to correct problems early, before they spoil the programme.

Selecting appropriate methods

It is not enough to decide what will be done, by whom and when, we also need to decide how it will be done.

In Chapter 1 some of the reasons for people's behaviour were discussed. Once a health worker understands the reasons behind behaviour that is causing a health problem, he or she can use many different methods to encourage a change in that behaviour. There are some important points to take into consideration when we choose a method. First of all, the method must suit the situation and the problem; it must therefore be selected carefully.

There are many methods, because there are many ways of solving a problem. Before choosing a method, the person practising health education must understand the problem at hand. A doctor, for example, has many methods to choose from in solving medical problems. If a patient is found to have a stomach ulcer, the doctor will try to understand the problem and choose the best method to use in dealing with it. If the ulcer is not too serious, diet may be the chosen method. By controlling what, when, and how much a person eats, the problem might be overcome. If the ulcer is slightly more serious, drugs may be used. In an even more serious case the doctor may choose to do an operation. It is likely that two or more methods will be used together.

People practising health education must make decisions about which methods should be used to help solve problems related to health behaviour. There are six things to consider before choosing health education methods:

● How ready and able are people to change?

● How many people are involved?

● Is the method appropriate to the local culture?

● What resources are available?

● What mixture of methods is needed?

● What methods fit the characteristics (age, sex, religion, etc.) of the target group?

How ready and able are people to change?

Remember the story in Chapter 1 about three women who were asked to buy shoes for their children. The midwife gave a talk in which she provided information, ideas, and suggestions. After the talk, not all the mothers decided to buy shoes.

One mother was ready to change. She had no major problems in her way. She accepted the ideas in the talk and carried out the midwife's suggestion. When people are ready to change, posters, radio, songs, plays, stories, displays, and photographs are some of the educational methods that can be used.

A second mother was interested in changing; she liked what the midwife had to say but she did not know if the family could spare the money for buying shoes. Also she was not sure if the grandmother would approve. The talk certainly gave this woman useful ideas about helping her children, but did not help her organize her family finances.

Approaches that might have helped this woman would have been discussion with family members about how much money they earned, how much they spent, and what they spent it on. Then, through demonstration or teaching, it might have been possible to show the family how to manage their money better so that shoes could be bought for the child. Linking the father with the local farmers' cooperative or with the agricultural extension agent might have helped him find ways of earning more money. Then if money was no longer a major problem, discussion with the grandmother about her love for her grandchild could have been used to win her support.

The third mother was hard to reach. She was so worried about her problems that it was difficult for her to take an interest in what the midwife said. She also lacked money and resources. To reach this woman, the midwife needed to use methods that allowed personal contact: counselling and home visits were needed. These would have shown the woman that the midwife was concerned, and would have helped the midwife to learn more about the woman's problems. The more she was able to learn, the more she would have been able to help.

This woman might have benefited from belonging to a group or club in which people with similar problems can support and encourage each other. Links with other community agencies could have provided the resources needed to help her care for her child. She could also have been helped by training in skills that would enable her to earn more money to provide for her child.

How many people are involved?

Some methods of health education are designed for reaching a large number of people (for example a group, a neighbourhood or a town) with a message or idea. These methods involve the use of such means as posters, lectures, displays, plays, role-plays, puppet shows, newspapers, radio, films, and town criers.

Providing good ideas quickly to a large number of people is a very useful step in health education. It creates awareness of a problem or idea. If the message is a good one, it will help prepare people to participate in desired action. However, other methods are usually needed to follow up the initial impression made through the mass media. Sending out health messages alone is usually not enough to change health behaviour in a large number of people.

In order to make large-group methods more useful in health education, there needs to be an exchange of views and ideas between the health or community workers who use the methods, and the people who see and hear the health messages. This exchange of views and ideas is called 'interaction'.

You will probably not be working alone. Share the responsibility of interacting with the community with other health workers, particularly with community health workers and staff from other community agencies.

Here are some suggestions for developing such interaction:

- After a film or talk, divide the audience into smaller groups for discussion.

- When putting up posters around the community, make home visits and discuss the ideas on the posters with families.

- After a play, ask the actors to go into the audience to talk with people.

- Organize small groups, in various parts of the community, for radio listening combined with discussion.

- Work with an existing community council or, if one does not exist, organize a community health committee (see pages 180–183).

Activities such as practising new skills, discussing personal feelings, values and money matters, and sharing difficult experiences are best done person-to-person or in small groups (ideally in, groups of no more than ten people).

Methods suitable for use with groups include story-telling, demonstrations, role-playing, case studies, discussions, educational games, and others that will be discussed in Chapter 5.

Teaching aids such as projectors and flip-charts may be used with groups of up to 25 people, although again it should be remembered that, when there are too many people, there will be

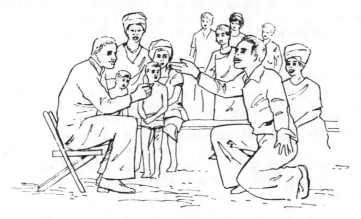

Role-playing can help individuals and small groups of people understand their problems and work out solutions to them. Some members of the group act out a situation, while others watch and make comments and suggestions.

less interaction and personal contact between the health worker and the members of the group.

Note that posters, radio, and other media designed to reach large groups can also be used with a small number of people.

Is the method appropriate to the local culture?

In Chapter 1 we described culture as the way of life of people in a community. Culture will determine the educational methods that will be acceptable and understandable to people. It will also determine the methods to which people will respond by changing to healthier behaviour.

For example, the role-playing method requires people to speak out freely in front of others. In one culture people may like to act and speak out. In another they may prefer to be quiet and careful about what they do or say. Role-playing would work well in the first culture. It may work in the second, but only after people in the group know and trust each other.

To take another example, photographs have different meanings in different cultures. If you are working in a community where most people are illiterate, they may not be used to seeing photos as a source of news or information, because they have little experience of books and newspapers. If you are doing a programme on breast-feeding in such a community, and show the women a picture of a mother breast-feeding her baby, their first thought may be that the photo is of your mother or sister. They would not realize that the photo is there to help them learn. Similar problems may arise in using films. We must make sure that people understand why they are being shown photographs or a film.

Role-playing and the use of photographs and films are examples of methods that will not work unless they are adapted to the culture of the community. Ways of adapting methods to culture are mentioned in Chapter 7. But we do not need to worry about adapting methods if we use some of the means by which the people themselves communicate ideas and share knowledge and skills. These include proverbs, town criers, plays, and so on. Such forms of natural communication should be part of any educational programme.

Practical demonstrations are good ways of teaching skills. In a good demonstration people will be given the chance to practise new skills.

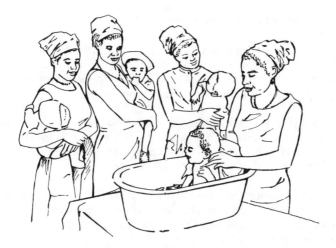

Instead of just talking about hygiene, this health worker is showing mothers how to bath their children.

What resources are needed?

Consider the resources necessary. Some methods require only yourself and the people around you: these include the use of stories and songs, role-playing, group discussions, and community meetings.

Other methods require the use of materials or teaching aids such as posters, flannelgraphs, demonstrations, models, puppet shows, newspapers, and flip-charts.

Then there are methods that use machines: tape recorders, film or slide projectors, etc. Machines usually need electricity. Machines and materials cost money. Try to look for methods that are inexpensive and at the same time effective.

Even if you are able to borrow films, projectors, and an electricity-generating plant, the films may come from a country whose culture your people will not understand. They may not even be in the language of your people. If that should be the case, a wiser decision would be to put on a play. A play simply needs people and a few materials. The local language can be used, and members of the community have a chance to participate. Expensive machines are not required.

Think of other ways in which you can use local resources to make or provide aids to education.

What mixture of methods is needed?

Select a mixture of methods. Variety and repetition are both important. By using a variety of methods you will make your programme more interesting. If you repeat the ideas in different ways, people are more likely to remember them.

If, for example, you are telling a story you may want to show some pictures or posters that relate to the story. Then after the story, you may ask some of the listeners to do a role-play in which they act out the story for all to see.

A health talk should be more than just talk. Of course, you will do some lecturing, but you should also show posters. There should be group discussion. Demonstrations and practice will also help people learn more from the talk.

A community meeting can be made more lively if a short play is also presented. This will help make issues more clear to people. A display could be added too. People coming to the meeting could look at the display and learn something about the subject before the meeting starts.

Which methods fit the group best?

You will meet different people and groups. Some will be old, some young. Some will be made up of women, some only of men, and some will be mixed. Select and adapt your methods to fit the type of people you meet.

Fables using animals might be better for children than for adults. Lectures may be better for educated people, than for those who have never been to school. If the people belong to one religion, select proverbs from the scriptures and books of that religion.

Evaluating results

If you have given time and effort to a project, you will want to know if it has been successful. In judging success, it is not enough simply to say 'we were very successful', or 'we had some success', or 'we failed'. If possible, a specific measure of the amount of success is needed.

Checking on the progress made

Observation, interviews, and records will supply information for evaluating a programme. Refer back to pages 71–73, that

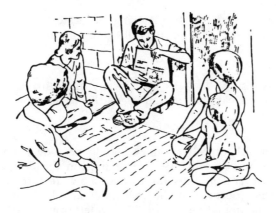

It is important to select the method (or methods) most appropriate for the group concerned. It is also important to use a mixture of methods that will help people to understand better and to remember.

show how a timetable can help a community in measuring progress as a community water supply programme develops. To take an example: it has been planned that the funds for the water supply project will be raised by the 12th week. If not enough money has been collected by that time, then something is wrong. The planning group must start to check and find the cause. Maybe the neighbourhood leaders were not adequately informed about how to organize fund-raising. Maybe it was a bad time of year for people to donate money because the harvest was not yet in.

If the plans were to dig four wells within six months, but only one is under way by the 17th or 18th week, then the group should immediately try to find out why. Maybe more materials are needed than originally planned. Maybe some of the labourers misunderstood their instructions.

Problems should be corrected as soon as they are seen.

Final results

By the end of the educational activities, you should be able to measure their success by counting how many people are behaving according to the original objectives: is this number more than before the programme started?

Use observation to check results. With community wells, for instance: is there evidence that they are maintained hygienically? Are people keeping them covered? Are they using clean buckets for gathering water? Are they storing the water in clean, covered containers at home? Are people still going to the stream to fetch water?

If people are using the wells hygienically and storing water safely at home, the educational objectives of the programme have been achieved.

As for the health objectives, there should be a decrease in the amount of waterborne disease. Depending on the type of disease, it may take several months for this to show. If a reduction in illness does not occur, test the well-water and look for other sources of contamination. If, in fact, waterborne disease is decreasing, then the programme has been successful.

Learning from evaluation

At the end of the programme, a final meeting can be held to discuss how far the programme has succeeded. Two main questions must be answered:

1. Did the action go as well as planned?

- Did people participate?

- Were resources available on time?

- Did people gain new skills and learn from the programme?

2. Was the problem eliminated or reduced? Using the example of schistosomiasis:

- Do people now have access to safe water supplies?

- Are people disposing of faeces and urine in a safe manner?

- Are fewer people suffering from the disease now than before the programme started?

Discussing such questions will help people evaluate and learn from their programmes. We can obtain the answers to these questions in the way in which we originally gathered information about the community when we started planning—through observation, interview, and records. Compare information gathered before the programme started with information collected after it ended.

Even if the programme did not turn out as desired, a meeting should still be held to find out why. A review of the timetable will help show if every person carried out his or her duties.

Questions such as these might help:

Were there any unreported difficulties earlier in the programme? Did other community events disturb or distract people from participating in the action? Were there any disagreements among community members that stopped them working together? Was the time set for the programme unrealistic? Were the activities chosen inappropriate to the local culture?

Once sources of difficulty have been found, the group can decide if it wants to try again. Learning can come from mistakes as well as from successes. It is a hopeful sign if people can sit down maturely and work out the cause of a problem. At such times, a health worker can provide much-needed support and encouragement. With new knowledge about the problem, the group will know how to plan a better programme in the future.

Reviewing the process of planning

We have seen the different steps that are involved in planning health education activities in primary health care. You will have noticed that, at each step, the health worker uses health education approaches that facilitate and reinforce the involvement of communities in health development. Through that involvement, you can make sure that the technology used is appropriate.

Using appropriate technology

Appropriate technology is an important factor for the success of primary health care. The word 'technology', as employed here, means an association of methods, techniques, and equipment which, together with the people using them, can contribute significantly to solving a health problem.

'Appropriate' technology means that, besides being scientifically sound, the technology is also acceptable to those who apply it and to those for whom it is used. This implies that technology should be in keeping with the local culture. It must be capable of being adapted and further developed if necessary.

In addition, the technology should be easily understood and applied by community health workers, and even by members of the community; although different forms of technology are appropriate at different stages of development, simplicity is always desirable. The most productive approach for ensuring that appropriate technology is available is to start with the problem and then to seek, or if necessary develop, technology that is relevant to local conditions and resources.

Involving the people in health care

The report of a WHO Expert Committee on New Approaches to Health Education in Primary Health Care[1] states that:

'to involve people and to enable them to formulate their own health care objectives, the health care providers will have to:

(*a*)   provide opportunities for people to learn how to identify and analyse health and health-related problems, and how to set their own targets;

(*b*)   make health and health-related information easily accessible to the community, including information on practical, effective, safe, and economical ways of attaining good health and of coping with disease and disability;

(*c*)   indicate to the people alternative solutions for solving the health and health-related problems they have identified;

(*d*)   create awareness of the importance of effective communication in fostering mutual understanding and support between the people and the health care providers;

(*e*)   translate the targets set by the people into simple, understandable, realistic, and acceptable goals which the communities can then monitor; and

(*f*)   help people to learn how to set priorities among the different health problems they have identified and to understand the need to refer to relevant policies in doing so, e.g., that priority should be given to the deprived sections of the community and to certain diseases on the basis of the degree of their contagiousness, susceptibility to treatment, etc.'

The report adds:

'It is essential that communities have a clear understanding of their role in the implementation of strategies for solving health problems. Here, health education should facilitate the dialogue with the people through culturally and socially acceptable forms of communication.'

[1] WHO Technical Report Series, No. 690, 1983.

Developing a partnership with the community

The subject of the Technical Discussions[1] held in May 1983 on the occasion of the Thirty-sixth World Health Assembly was 'New policies for health education in primary health care'. More than 300 delegates to the Assembly took part. They discussed the need to develop a real partnership between health workers and the community at every stage of health planning, from identifying problems, through facilitating and reinforcing health action, to evaluating results. There should be a constant dialogue and inter-action between the community and the health workers.

People may 'feel' many health and related problems, but they may not be able to express them clearly. There may be other major problems that they do not see. The health worker should encour-age and guide the community in self-study so that the community can better understand its problems, identify local resources to solve them, and call on outside help when needed.

As action to solve a problem is developed, the health worker will assist the community in examining whether its efforts are worthwhile and effective. Are the desired changes occurring in the community? Have obstacles to progress arisen? Are the chosen technologies and strategies appropriate? In other words, the health worker should involve the community in a constant cycle of planning, action, and evaluation. By encouraging involvement and continuous self-examination, the health worker will be educating the community about the planning process. This makes future self-help efforts possible.

The chart on pages 86–87 illustrates how a real partnership between health workers and the community can develop.

Coordinating levels of planning

Coordination is an important job in health education. We need to provide a link between people and the various resource agencies and to foster communication between the people and the agencies. We should also encourage communication among the agencies themselves so that they will make the most effective use of their resources in assisting the community. We must also be aware that this assistance will come from different levels—district, regional, state, and national.

---

[1] Each year, the Member States of the World Health Organization assemble in Geneva to determine the policies of the Organization and take action to further the objectives of WHO. On this occasion Technical Discussions are held on specified subjects of international interest. This was the second time that health education was the subject of the Technical Discussions: the first time was in 1958.

Decentralized functions

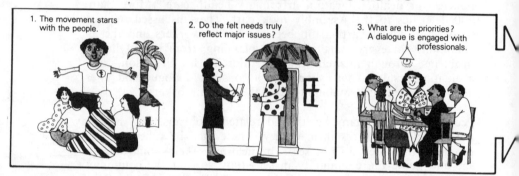

Information and education fo

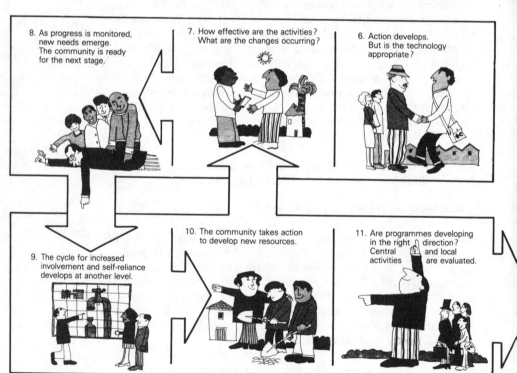

Centralized functions

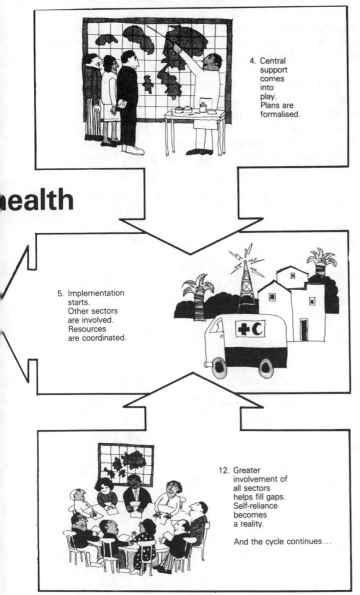

ealth

4. Central support comes into play. Plans are formalised.

5. Implementation starts. Other sectors are involved. Resources are coordinated.

12. Greater involvement of all sectors helps fill gaps. Self-reliance becomes a reality.

And the cycle continues...

This chart shows how a real partnership develops between health workers and the community through the various stages of identifying problems, then facilitating and reinforcing health action. This chart was developed in connection with the Technical Discussions on 'New policies for health education in primary health care' at the Thirty-sixth World Health Assembly in May 1983.

Primary health care is a national concern, not just a local one. Ministries and agencies at the central level are also planning for the effective delivery of primary health care services. It is necessary for the community to be aware of these central planning efforts so that it may benefit from the resources. An example of a central function would be the supply of essential drugs to all communities. Another important central function of direct relevance to health education is the planning of mass media (radio, television, etc.) programmes on priority health needs.

The community and health workers together must make sure that their needs for essential drugs, basic transportation, educational media, and other resources are constantly communicated to the central planning authorities. Likewise the central planners must always be in touch with local communities to hear their needs and thereby be in a better position to plan for primary health care.

Chapter 4

Health education with individuals

Counselling is one of the approaches most frequently used in health education to help individuals and families.

During counselling, a person with a need and a person who provides support and encouragement (the counsellor) meet and discuss in such a way that the person with a need gains confidence in his or her ability to find solutions to the problems. Counselling relies heavily on communication and relationship skills.

Opportunities for counselling arise whenever we work with individuals and families: with patients at the health centre, with pupils at school, or during a home visit, to name a few. Counselling should be part of the treatment and care given to a sick or troubled person. It is also an important aspect of disease prevention and health promotion because it helps people to understand what they can do, through their own efforts, to avoid illness and to improve their lives.

This chapter describes:

- The purpose of counselling (pages 89–90).

- The rules to follow when acting as a counsellor (pages 90–92).

- The different types of counselling (pages 92–97).

- Ways to facilitate decisions and follow-through (pages 97–101).

- A sample counselling session (pages 101–106).

- Suggestions for practice in counselling (pages 106–107).

The purpose of counselling

Through counselling, individuals are encouraged to think about their problems and thus come to a greater understanding of the causes. As a result of this understanding people will, it is hoped, commit themselves to taking action that will solve the problems. The kind of action taken will be a person's own decision, although it may be guided, if necessary by the counsellor.

Counselling means choice, not force, not advice. A health worker may think that his or her advice seems reasonable, but it may not be appropriate to the particular circumstances of the person receiving the advice. With counselling, it is the person concerned who takes the decisions so that the solutions adopted are more likely to be appropriate. An appropriate solution will be one that the person can follow with successful results.

Here is an example of the problems that arise when a person is advised and forced:

> During a home visit one health worker saw a mother with three-week-old twins. The babies were so small that the health worker worried that they might not live. She scolded the mother for not coming to the clinic.
>
> The health worker advised the mother to come to the hospital with the twins immediately and stay there with them until they became bigger and stronger. The mother nodded her head in agreement. While she was packing her things, she began to cry.
>
> A brother of the woman's husband came to see what she was crying about. The health worker explained, but the man became angry. He said there were many good reasons why the woman was crying. She was worried because, if she stayed in hospital, there would be no one to care for her other two children. She had recently moved to another town with her husband. She felt that there would be no one whom her children knew and trusted enough to stay with. Also the mother was crying for fear that the health worker might refuse to help her in the future, if she did not agree to go to hospital now.

Rules for counselling

The health worker in this example had obviously not learned the techniques of counselling, otherwise she would have followed the simple rules below.

Relationships

Counsellors show concern and a caring attitude. They pay attention to building a good relationship from the beginning with the person they are trying to help. People are more likely to talk about their problems with someone they trust.

Identifying needs

Counsellors seek to understand a problem as the person with the problem sees it. People must identify their own problems.

90

Counsellors do not name the problems for them. The use of questions that lead to open comments will help here (see page 50). A counsellor's task is to listen carefully.

Feelings

Counsellors develop empathy (understanding and acceptance) for a person's feelings, not sympathy (sorrow or pity). A counsellor would never say 'You should not worry so much about that.' It is natural for people to have worries and fears about their problems. A good counsellor helps people to become aware of their feelings and to cope with them.

Participation

Counsellors never try to persuade people to accept their advice. If the advice turns out to be wrong, the person will be angry and no longer trust the counsellor. If the advice is right, the person may become dependent on the counsellor for solving all problems.

Counsellors help people to think about all the factors involved in their problems, and encourage people to choose the solutions that are best in their particular situation.

Secrecy

Counsellors will be told about many personal and possibly embarrassing problems. The information must be kept secret from all other people, even from the client's relatives. If a person you are counselling discovers that you have told other people about the counselling session, that person will no longer trust you and will avoid you. A client may even get into trouble because of what a counsellor has told others. Counsellors always respect the privacy of the people they are helping. They never reveal information without specific permission.

Information and resources

Although counsellors do not give advice, they should share information and ideas on resources which the client needs in order to make a sound decision. For example, many people do not realize the connection between their behaviour and their health. Counsellors do not lecture, but should provide simple facts during discussion to help people have a clearer view of their problems.

All health or community workers can practise a counselling approach in their work. Parents and friends can be counsellors too. The important thing is that the nurse, teacher, father, or friend is willing to listen carefully and encourage the person to take as much responsibility as possible for solving his or her own problem.

> Now that you have read about the rules for counselling, think again about the case of the mother with twins. How could the health worker have made a better beginning with this home visit? What comments and questions could have been used to find out more about the mother's problems? How could the other relatives in the house have been involved? Can you think of possible alternative solutions to the problem?

Different types of counselling

Counselling with families

People may need the help of their families to solve a problem. Counselling skills are useful whether the counsellor is working with one person or with a whole family.

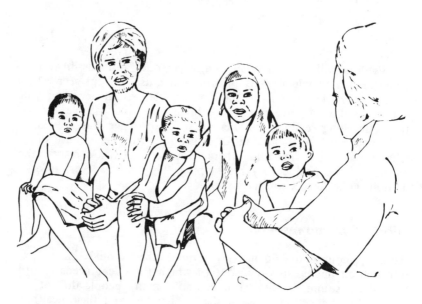

Sometimes it is necessary to involve the whole family in solving a health problem. Remember that each member of the family has different responsibilities in the home and therefore can help, in different ways, to find solutions.

When working with a family, we are dealing with more than one person, therefore there may be more than one problem, more than one need, and probably more than one solution.Also, be aware that in families different people have different responsibilities and powers. The father, for example, may have the major say on how money is spent by the family. The mother may make most of the decisions about the types of food eaten. Grandparents influence the degree to which families follow traditional customs. Find and talk to the right person for each problem. Also, show respect to the recognized head of the household.

Counselling with children

In a clinic, a school, or the community, you will find children with health, emotional, or other problems. Counselling can be provided for them if they are old enough to talk.

It is better to talk to the child alone. Background information can be obtained from the parents first; then they can be politely asked to wait outside. Sometimes parents want to answer all the questions; they do not give the child a chance to speak. The child may also be afraid of saying certain things in front of parents. The counsellor should explain to the parents that the child may speak more freely without others around.

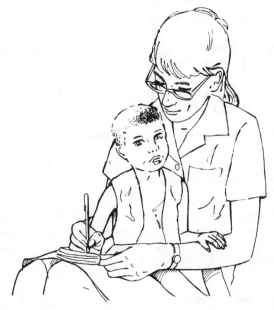

This health worker is holding a child. This inspires confidence and trust. Now the child is willing to talk to the health worker about his problems.

Begin by talking about happy things. Ask the child about his or her favourite games, for example. Once the child is relaxed, begin talking about the problem. Let the child know that everything said will be kept secret. In this way the child will trust you and speak freely. Always keep your promise of secrecy. If parents, teachers, or others find out what has been said, the child will be afraid, and never let the counsellor help again.

Follow the counselling rules with a child as you would with an adult. The child will be able to learn much about health from a good counsellor.

Home visits

Counselling can be done in the clinic or at school, but home visits are also helpful. Health workers should visit all homes in their communities regularly. If a village is small, with 10–25 houses, visits can be made at least once a fortnight. In larger villages or neighbourhoods, visits can be made monthly. Here are some reasons for home visits:

- Keeping a good relationship with people and families.

- Encouraging the prevention of common diseases.

- Detecting and improving troublesome situations early, before they become big problems.

- Checking on the progress of a sick person, or on progress towards solving other problems.

- Educating the family on how to help a sick person.

- Informing people about important community events in which their participation is needed.

Much can be learned from home visits. We can see how the environment and the family situation might affect a person's behaviour. Does the family have resources such as a well? Which relatives stay in the house? Do they help or hinder the person's progress?

When people are in their own homes, they usually feel happier and more secure. You may find that people are more willing to talk in their own homes than when they are at the clinic. At the

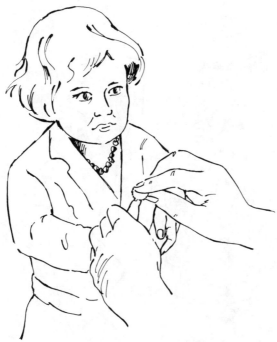

Children are often afraid when they are sick. Before a health worker can treat and counsel a child, he or she must gain the child's trust and make the child feel comfortable.

clinic they may fear that other people will see them or overhear the discussion. They may tell more at home, because they feel safer there.

Nutrition demonstrations, for example, may be more useful if done in a person's home. There the health worker will be able to use the exact materials and facilities that the person must use. This will make the demonstration more realistic and make learning easier. In Chapter 5 we will examine the organization of such demonstrations.

If you approach people with understanding, they will welcome you into their homes. There you will find many opportunities for health education.

When was the last time you made a home visit? What was the reason? Did the people welcome you? If people seemed afraid, what can you do next time to improve the relationship?

Did you use counselling in that home? How did the people respond? How can you make a better home visit next time?

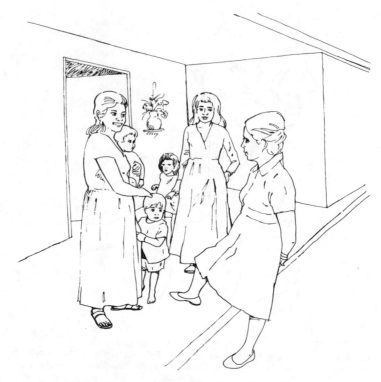

During a home visit, a health worker can check on the progress of a sick person, meet other family members who can help care for the patient, observe new problems, and encourage preventive action.

Educational methods used in counselling

There are various educational methods that can be used to help individuals and families solve their problems. Some help people understand the cause of their problem. Some help them see possible solutions, while other methods help them reach decisions for action.

We have seen in Chapters 1 and 3 how important it is for us to place ourselves in the position of other people and understand why they behave as they do. But the people themselves also need to see why there is a problem. Our role therefore is first to understand the problem, and then to help the people understand it themselves. Next we need to work together with them to find solutions that are appropriate to their situations.

Sometimes people may be reluctant to take the action necessary to solve their problems. They may not feel that it is worth the time and effort. Encourage them to examine their values in order to take some decision about the importance they place on their health and welfare.

Another way to help people decide to act is the use of self-reward. People should decide on a reward that they will give themselves if they follow through with the necessary action. We will discuss this idea on pages 100–101.

It is important to help people choose solutions that will fit in with their ways of doing things, and with their beliefs. Try to help them avoid solutions that are uncomfortable. Find workable alternatives.

It may also be helpful to link a person with someone who has successfully coped with a similar problem as in the following example.

> Mrs Angelino has recently learned that she has diabetes. She is worried about how she will manage the changes in her diet and activities and how she will test her urine and take her drugs. The health worker decided it would be helpful to introduce Mrs Angelino to Mrs Pedro who has been on diabetes treatment for five years. Mrs Pedro can provide support and encouragement based on her own personal experience.

Always remember that counselling calls essentially for a personal approach and for skills in listening, in providing information, and in helping people themselves determine what is best for them.

Demonstrating and displaying real objects are educational methods that can be used to counsel an individual.

Facilitating decisions and follow-through

What are the things we value most?

As we said in Chapter 1, values are standards and beliefs that are very important to us and that therefore affect our behaviour. Some of the things people value include progress, happiness, friendship, security, and comfort. If asked, most people would say that they value health, but too often they do not think about their health until they have lost it.

Although people feel strongly about their values, they do not always seem to behave in ways that match them. People often do not even realize that the way they are behaving is not consistent with their values. The examples below show this clearly.

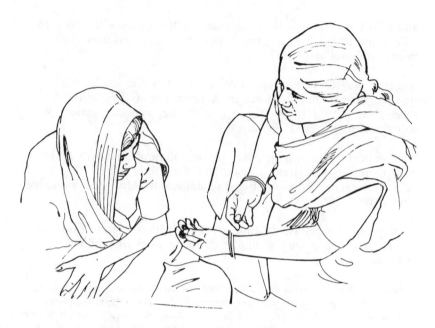

This health worker is counselling a woman on family planning methods.

People value their children very highly. They consider it an honour to be a parent. Caring for children is a special duty not to be taken lightly. But sometimes you see a family spending their extra money on new clothing, cigarettes, or alcohol, even though the children are underweight and sickly. It may be that the family wants new clothing so that they can all feel proud when they attend a relative's marriage. Maybe they drink alcohol because their friends do or because it seems a way to help them mix easily with other people. Maybe they believe cigarettes will help them concentrate better at their work. Perhaps the family does not know that children need to eat certain foods to be healthy. You can probably think of other reasons for this family's behaviour. It is unlikely that the mother and father want to hurt their children. They probably do not realize that their behaviour is out of line with the value they place on their children.

Look now at the example of a schoolboy who has an infected toe. He complains a lot about the pain. He says he values his health. The health worker tells him to come to the clinic for injections for five days. After the second day, the boy does not come again. There are many possible reasons for this. Maybe the pain has been relieved and he thinks two injections are enough. Maybe it is a long way to the clinic. Maybe the boy has important work or ah examination at school. He may be afraid of the health worker or the injections. Whatever the reason, the boy probably does not see that his behaviour is working against his stated value of health.

> Clarify your own values. You may have to think hard. What are the five things you value most in life? Now look at one of them. Think back over the past week. Have you always behaved in a way that is in line with the value selected? If not, for what reasons? Why is it difficult for people always to behave according to their values? What can you do to bring your own behaviour more in line with your values?

Adjusting behaviour to values

It is our role to help people see clearly how their values may not be matched by their behaviour. Then perhaps, they will try to change. If they are to do so, we need to help them find out what matters most in their lives. This is best done with individuals, although it can also be done in small groups. Values are very personal. People are unlikely to talk in front of others about their values and the contradictions in their behaviour.

The discussions of this topic would usually be part of an individual counselling session. You would already have found out some of the problems the client is facing, and some of the reasons for these problems. Begin by asking what the client sees as the most important things in life—what is valued most. Ask what the client does to live up to these values. If health is valued, what does the client do to keep healthy? If children are valued, what does the client do to make sure children grow up to be strong and successful?

Once people are clear about the things they value most in life, ask them if they always act in ways that are in harmony with their values. If they say 'No', ask them why. Find out what makes it difficult for them to live always according to their values. Also if you have noticed any differences in the values a person holds and the person's actions, gently point them out. The realization of such differences is a very important step towards the decision to change one's behaviour. But once a person has decided to modify certain habits, that decision has to be kept to day after day, until the changes in behaviour have become part of a way of life. This is often very difficult. We will see now how people can be strengthened in their decision to adopt healthy practices.

Using self-rewards

If people receive a benefit for an action, they will be encouraged or motivated to repeat that action. Rewards can encourage good health behaviour. But they must be used with caution. First, they should be used only when a form of behaviour is very difficult to change (for example, cigarette-smoking).

Secondly, a health worker should be aware that it is quite possible to mislead someone by using rewards and thus cause many problems. To avoid this, always make sure, first, that people choose the kind of healthy behaviour that they want to achieve and, second, that they choose their own rewards. Otherwise a problem like the following may result.

> Mr Tem has hypertension. He is supposed to come to the clinic once a month to have his blood pressure checked and his supply of medicaments renewed. Unfortunately, Mr Tem comes to the clinic only when he is feeling unwell.
>
> The physician on duty is worried about Mr Tem. He tells him that he will give him the money for his transport if he comes every month. Mr Tem agrees and begins coming to the clinic regularly.
>
> Several months later the physician is transferred to another hospital. When Mr Tem meets the new physician, he asks for his transport money. The physician is surprised and says that he cannot afford to give patients money every month. Mr Tem is angry at this. Since that day he has not returned to the clinic. When he feels unwell, he buys drugs from a local drug-seller.

In the above example, the first physician failed to help Mr Tem, because the physician made all the choices. In health education, people must choose to change their own behaviour and choose the rewards they will give themselves if they are successful. It is also important to try other methods first. If Mr Tem was having money problems, a better method would have been to link him with a social welfare agency.

Here is an example of how a health worker encouraged her client to participate in choosing self-rewards.

> Mr Solo had been coughing for some years. The health worker helped Mr Solo understand that cigarettes made him cough more. When he understood this, he said he wanted to stop smoking. He tried to cut down, but by the next week he was smoking as much as before. He came back to the health worker for help.
>
> The health worker listened to Mr Solo. She agreed that he was having a difficult time. She asked Mr Solo to tell her some of the things he liked to do in his free time. He said he really enjoyed playing draughts with his

neighbour. She asked if he had any favourite foods. He said that chicken was his favourite, but that he could not afford to have it very often. His wife prepared chicken only once or twice a month.

The health worker then explained the idea of rewards to Mr Solo. She said that he could reward himself with something he liked, if he stopped smoking. Mr Solo thought about this. Then he said he would talk to his wife and his neighbour. On days when he did not smoke a cigarette, he would play draughts with the neighbour; if he smoked, he would stay at home and not play. He liked draughts very much, so playing would be a reward. While playing, the neighbour could help to remind Mr Solo not to smoke. (Support from friends and relatives is another important factor in health education.) Also, he would put aside the money saved by not smoking and give it to his wife so that she would make him a chicken dinner as a reward.

Finally, rewards should be something that is good for the person. A child may say 'I want candy if I clean my teeth every day.' Eating candy every day is not very healthy for a child. Maybe a small amount of candy at the end of the week would be possible. Better still, find another reward.

Compare the examples of Mr Tem and Mr Solo. In which case was the health worker correct in using rewards? Can you think of better ways to encourage Mr Tem to attend the clinic without using rewards? Do you think Mr Solo will keep his promise to stop smoking? What other approaches might be used to help Mr Solo and Mr Tem?

A sample counselling session

Here is an example of a problem that requires counselling: A teacher has asked a community health worker to talk to one of his students. The teacher tells the community health worker several things about the student. He is seventeen years old. He is intelligent, but lately has missed a lot of time from school. He always seems tired. This is the student's final year, and the teacher is worried that he may not pass his exams.

The discussion that follows shows what the community health worker might do in this situation. Pay careful attention to what he says. Note that he asks general questions to start the boy talking freely. He greets the boy and tries to build up a good relationship. He listens carefully to all that the boy says. No advice is given until the community health worker has heard the whole story behind the boy's problem.

Also the community health worker encourages the boy to think carefully about the problem so that he can understand the cause better and come up with some possible solutions for himself. Remember that people are more committed to solving their problems if they participate in developing the solutions.

If you are with other people, you can use this counselling session as a short play. Ask everyone to read the discussion once. Get two volunteers. One will read aloud the part of the community health worker, the other will read aloud what the boy says. This will be a good way to practise counselling.

Sample counselling session

Health worker:	Good morning. I hope everything is going well with you and your parents.
Boy:	Thank you. Everyone is all right except that Mother has some back trouble.
Health worker:	I believe that this is your last year at school. How are your studies coming along?
Boy:	Well, I usually do fine at school, but you know the last year is always difficult.
Health worker:	Have you been healthy so far this year?
Boy:	Actually, I've been feeling a bit weak and get these headaches. I thought it was probably malaria, but I am not sure.
Health worker:	Malaria is bad at this time of year. Did you take any medicine for it?
Boy:	I've taken the full course of chloroquine tablets about three times so far, but I never seem to get completely well.
Health worker:	The tablets are necessary, but medicine alone cannot solve all our problems. Are you eating well?
Boy:	I think so.
Health worker:	Tell me, what have you been taking for your meals the past few days?
Boy:	My mother always tells us to have a good breakfast, so I make big bowls of cereal for myself and my brothers. Then, too, I always try to buy fruit.
Health worker:	You are saying that you do some cooking and shopping?
Boy:	These jobs are necessary. A few years ago my mother hurt her back. Now it is giving her a lot of trouble. The doctor says she is getting older and there is not much

	more that can be done. They give her pain-relievers, but the doctor told all of us children to try to help our mother in any way possible. Since I am the oldest, most of the responsibility falls on me.
Health worker:	What other chores do you have?
Boy:	I help prepare the evening meal too. I get the smaller children to clean the house, but I have to watch them to see that they do it well.
Health worker:	With all this work, when do you find time to study?
Boy:	That is a problem. It is really hard to do any serious studying until the chores are done and the younger children have settled down for the night. Then I read for as many hours as possible, or until I just fall asleep at the table.
Health worker:	Where do you actually study?
Boy:	As you know, we only have two rooms to live in. One is my parents' bedroom. The other is used for sitting and eating in, and as the children's bedroom. That's why I can't concentrate on my studies until the younger ones are asleep. I even try not to turn the lamp up too bright so they won't wake and disturb me.
Health worker:	I can see that things are difficult for you just now. From what you have said, you are under a lot of stress. I realize that you have duties you must carry out for your family, but I think all this extra work and reading late at night in a poor light have contributed to your feeling of weakness and your headaches. Does this sound reasonable to you?
Boy:	I guess I never thought about it like that before, but it does make sense. I am worried, however. As you said, I do have to do my chores at home. How can I deal with this problem?
Health worker:	First, what do you really want to achieve?
Boy:	I want to pass my exams this year, so I probably need to study more.
Health worker:	And to be able to study more you have to be strong and rested.
Boy:	That's true, so I also have to figure out how to get more rest.
Health worker:	Let us think about when you might find more time to study. You say you prepare the evening meal and do some shopping. What do you do between the time you leave school and the time you start preparing the meal?
Boy:	Usually after school I walk to the market to pick up the few things I may need for the evening meal. There I meet some friends and we talk and play games for a

while. Then when I see the sun is going down, I go home to start the meal.

Health worker: Play is necessary to keep your body fit, but do you think it might be possible to spare some time after school a couple of days a week to do a little reading? Reading in daylight would be better on your eyes than reading by a dim lamp at night.

Boy: That makes sense. I really like playing with my friends, though.

Health worker: I am not saying that you should stop playing, because playing helps keep you fit. But you do have to think about what is most important to you. You do seem worried about your school work. You must decide for yourself what sacrifice you are ready to make for the sake of your studies. Right now you are sacrificing your health.

Boy: I never thought of it that way, but you are right, I do value my studies and, if I am not in good health, I cannot do well in school. I am sure I could stay after school an extra hour and read at my desk there. No one would disturb me then, and even the teachers might still be around. They could help me with any questions I had. My friends would not miss me for only one hour, so I could join them later. I hope they will not make fun of me for wanting to remain at school.

Health worker: Do your friends understand the problems you have at home?

Boy: Of course, they always stop by the house at the weekend to say "hello" to my mother and ask how she is. I guess they would understand and not make fun of me.

Health worker: Now about weekends. Can you arrange time to study then?

Boy: Saturday morning is usually taken up with chores. And after that the house is never quiet. The younger children are always running in and out and then there are visitors.

Health worker: Do you have to stay at home to study?

Boy: Maybe I could see if some of the classrooms at the school are open, or I could even go out to my father's farm. It is always quiet there. I could take some snacks and sit under those big shady trees.

Health worker: It's good that you are able to think of so many solutions to this problem. The teacher was right. You are a bright boy. Now I'm interested to know about your younger brothers. How old are they?

Boy: The next younger is thirteen, and then there are the twins aged nine.

Health worker: The one who is thirteen – is he also doing well at school?

Boy: He tries very hard. His grades have been almost as good as mine. He could probably do better.

Health worker: How old were you when your mother's back trouble began?

Boy: About fourteen.

Health worker: And you had to start doing all those chores from that age?

Boy: Yes.

Health worker: I was just thinking that if your brother is also a bright boy, and since he is nearly fourteen, maybe he could also start taking on more responsibility in the home. What do you think about this?

Boy: I have always thought of him as being very young, but, if I could handle the chores at his age, I am sure he could manage too. Maybe we could take turns with the cooking and other jobs. That would be another way for me to get more rest and more time for study.

Health worker: With all the ideas you have mentioned, I am sure you will have no more trouble with your studies, but please feel free to come to me again if you or any other member of your family has problems. Now, before you leave, please remind me of the things you are going to do to solve your problems. It will help us to make sure that we have forgotten nothing and that we are satisfied with what we have decided.

Boy: First I need to get more rest and find better times for study. I will stay after school for about an hour so I can read in the daylight. Then at weekends I will go to the farm to read. At home I will get my younger brother to take turns with me in doing the cooking and other chores.

Health worker: Thank you. That's very good. Now give my regards to your parents.

Boy: I will. Thank you for your help. Good bye.

In this example the health worker never assumed that he understood the boy's problem until he had enough information. He never forced the boy to take advice. He always encouraged the boy to think about his problem and make his own decisions.

He asked questions that helped the boy to think carefully and seriously about the cause of the problem.

When the health worker discovered that the boy was reluctant to give up his play time, he asked the boy to examine his values. The health worker helped the boy realize what things were really important to him and guided the boy in making choices. A compromise was then reached so that the boy could study more, but not give up playing with his friends.

More practice in counselling

Like any skill, counselling improves with practice. Gather some other health or community workers and do a role-play (see pages 152–157 in the next chapter for details on role-playing). One of you will be a counsellor. The other will be a mother whose child has an infected ear. The remaining people will be the audience. They have an important job: they should watch the role-play carefully and at the end they can give the players suggestions for improving their counselling skills.

Suggestions for the person who plays the role of the mother

You should behave just like a normal mother in your community. What might a mother believe is the cause of the illness? What local treatments might she have been using before coming to the clinic? The counsellor may be interested in the mother's family, living conditions, and occupation. Make up a story about yourself, so you can give realistic answers to the counsellor. You have watched mothers come to the clinic many times. Sometimes they are worried and afraid. Behave just like the mothers you have seen. That will make the role-play better.

Suggestions for the counsellor

Remember the simple counselling steps. Think of what educational tools you can use. Can you demonstrate a skill that needs to be learned by the mother? Could you use posters or pictures? You may not have these with you, but in a role-play you can pretend that you have them. Can you make up a story, proverb, or fable? Will you need to help the mother get support from family members?

Do not rush the counselling

It is natural for the session to go slowly at first. After you have had a lot of practice and real sessions, your skills will increase. You will be able to understand problems more quickly and select educational methods more easily.

For further practice, use the case of the mother with twins (see page 90) as the basis for a role-play. People could take the roles of health worker, mother, brother-in-law, and possibly other relatives. Also you should make up your own role-plays based on actual problem situations you have seen in the clinic, school, and community. Always have a few other people watch the plays so that they can suggest improvements.

Whatever the situation may be, remember that counselling implies the following four steps:

1. Helping the client identify what is the problem.

2. Helping the client discover why it is a problem.

3. Encouraging the client to look at many possible solutions to the problem.

4. Having the client choose the most appropriate solution.

Chapter 5

Health education with groups

Working with groups is a major activity in health education. When people get together to identify, define, and solve a problem, they have many more resources than when they work individually. Groups can often do things that several individuals could not do by themselves. Groups support their members in the practice of health behaviour. They also enable people to learn from each other.

This chapter first considers:

- What is a group? (pages 108–109).

- Formal groups and informal gatherings (pages 109–111).

- People's behaviour in formal groups (pages 111–114).

Then, after a discussion of the value of group education (page 114), health education methods in relation to the following groups are dealt with in some detail:

- Informal groups or gatherings (pages 115–124).

- Formal groups or associations (pages 125–128).

- Discussion groups (pages 128–131).

- Self-help groups (pages 131–134).

- The school classroom (pages 134–140).

- Health education at the work-site (pages 140–158).

- Demonstrations (pages 144–147).

- Case studies (pages 147–152).

- Role-playing (pages 152–157).

- A group training session (pages 158–159).

- The health team (pages 160–163).

- Conducting meetings (pages 163–170).

Each group has a personality of its own. Each group also has a different potential for action. To work effectively with a group, it is important to use the methods that are best suited to that group.

What is a group?

As used in this manual, the word 'group' may be defined as a gathering of two or more people who have a common interest.

Here are examples of the groups often found in a community:

- A family
- A council of village elders.
- People working at the same factory, business, or agency.
- A class of schoolchildren.
- A farmers' cooperative.
- People attending a religious ceremony together.
- A women's association.

- A youth club.
- An association or guild of craftsmen.
- Some friends getting together to relax.
- People riding together on a bus.
- A gathering of patients at a clinic.

Formal groups and informal gatherings

There are two main kinds of group. Those that are very well organized, such as farmers' cooperatives, are formal groups. Those that are not organized, such as the people attending market on a particular day, are informal gatherings.

The following are some characteristics of formal groups.

- A formal group has a purpose or goal that everyone in the group knows, accepts, and tries to achieve by working together with the others.

- There is a set membership, so people know who belongs and who does not.

- There are recognized leaders (group members who have the special responsibility of guiding the group towards achievement of its goals).

- There are organized activities such as regular meetings and projects.

- The group has rules that members agree to follow.

- Attention is paid to the welfare of the members.

The people in an informal gathering have some feature in common, but no special goal that they are trying to achieve together. For example, most of those attending a preschool clinic are women (with their children); their common feature is that they are mothers and that each is concerned about her child. Of course, once the group is assembled at the clinic, it may set out to accomplish a certain task, perhaps one suggested by the health worker.

The following are some characteristics of informal gatherings.

- There is no special membership or feeling of belonging.

- People come and go at will.

- While people of importance in the community may be at the gathering, it has no special leader. In fact leadership may come from outside the group. For example, the nurse at a clinic may provide leadership to a gathering of patients.

- Usually no special activity is planned by the people themselves; like people coming to watch a football match, everyone just happens to be in the same place at the same time.

- No special rules apply.

- There is usually more concern for self, and less for the welfare of the other people present.

The purpose of formal groups

Formal groups fulfil two major needs:

The need to accomplish a task

In most formal groups people work together to plan projects, organize activities, and solve problems. A farming cooperative may be working towards buying some new farm tools. A social club may be planning a party for the next holiday. People choose to work in groups because tasks can be accomplished more easily if several people work together.

The need to belong

Human beings want to feel that other people like them and accept them. People also want respect from others. One reason why people come together in groups is to get a feeling of being liked, accepted, and respected by others.

A group is successful if it can meet both of these needs for its members. If a group can never solve a problem or plan a programme, members will lose interest and leave. If people in the group are not friendly, always argue, or ignore the welfare of other members, there will not be much feeling of belonging. A successful group will make people feel welcome and at the same time accomplish tasks in a cooperative way.

Name as many formal groups as you can think of in your community. Do you know the purpose or goal of each group? Who are the leaders? What does one have to do, or be, to become a member? Can you tell who is a member and who is not? What are some of the organized activities of those groups? Do you know any of the rules the groups have for their members?

Name some informal groups or gatherings in your community? What common features do people in these groups share? Are there common interests that could form the basis of an educational programme?

Behaviour in formal groups

It is the behaviour of individual members that helps make a group a success or failure. Let us look at two quite different examples of group behaviour and analyse them.

Problem behaviour

Consider this example:

The Unity Health Committee was formed two years ago. The members originally thought that, if they worked together, they could identify and solve some of the major health problems in the community. They had set the following priority goals for the year:

To increase attendance at the preschool clinics.

To double the number of children receiving immunization.

To make sure all mothers have road-to-health charts for their preschool children.

They have still not been able to achieve any of those goals.

During a meeting, the leader of the group says 'At our last meeting, only half the members were present. We cannot expect to achieve anything if our members are not serious about attending our meetings. Today we must decide on a way to improve clinic attendance. We can never hope to increase immunization coverage if mothers do not attend the clinics.'

Member A says 'I think we should borrow a loudspeaker van to inform mothers about the clinics.'

Member B answers 'That is a foolish idea. You know we would have to go to the district headquarters to request the van, and transport to the headquarters is very expensive.'

Member A decides to say no more. She feels bad because she was called foolish before everyone in the group. She makes no more suggestions during the rest of the meeting.

The leader asks if anyone has another idea. Member C suggests 'Let us go on house-to-house visits to encourage mothers to attend.'

Member B answers again 'That would take a lot of time, and you know all of us are busy with our own work. I had to leave my business to attend this meeting. Don't waste our time with silly ideas.'

Member C is angry. He says to Member B 'You always criticise other people's ideas. Why don't you suggest something better yourself?' Then the two of them start arguing. The leader, after 15 minutes, tries to calm them down. Member C and some of his friends finally get up and walk out of the meeting.

The behaviour of the members in this group is causing the group to fail. Member B talks too much. He always criticises. He does not add useful ideas. He makes other people feel bad. Member A gives up. If she is silent, she cannot contribute to solving the problem. Member C becomes angry too easily. Instead of facing the group's problems, he runs away. Other members do not show any interest; many do not attend. The leader lets members get deep into an argument before taking any action to stop them. Instead of encouraging them to resolve their differences right away, he allows them to fight.

Positive behaviour

Let us now see how people in the Progress Health Committee behave.

Last year the community faced a big problem when the main water-hole dried up for three months. The health committee is now holding a meeting to find a permanent solution to the water problem. The leader starts the meeting by saying 'I am glad to see that so many of you could come and that everyone is on time. We will be able to get a lot of work done today. I do not see Member D. Does anyone know where he is?'

'His wife is sick, so he took her to the clinic' says Member E. Then Member F suggests 'We should go to his house after the meeting and find out how his wife is.' Everyone agrees.

Then the leader reminds the group about their problem. He asks for suggestions for improving the community water supply. Member G suggests 'We could dig a large community well.'

Member H answers 'Thank you for your suggestion. A well could help if we can afford it. What is the opinion of our treasurer?'

The treasurer informs the group 'We are very short of money just now. I wish I knew where to find the money. Maybe Member J has an idea. She recently visited her uncle whose village has just finished building a deep new well.'

Member J replies 'The community development agents in my uncle's village told him about a special programme that gives loans to communities for self-help projects. Maybe we could get a loan too.'

'That's a good idea,' says Member E. 'I will volunteer to visit our own community development agent to see if he knows anything about loans.

What good behaviour did you notice in this group? Think first and then see (a) if you agree with the kinds of helpful behaviour listed below; (b) if you have any additions to the list:

Examples of helpful behaviour:

- Making suggestions.

- Encouraging each other to talk.

- Responding politely to the suggestions of others.

- Helping make points clear.

- Giving information.

- Showing concern for each other.

- Volunteering to help with work.

- Attending meetings regularly and on time.

- Thanking each other for suggestions given.

Conflict in groups

Disagreements are natural when people come together in groups. In both the Unity and Progress Health Committees there was some conflict or divergence of views about solutions to their problems. In the Unity Committee some people gave in without discussing their views fully. Some fought. Others ran away. Such behaviour is not helpful for solving problems.

In the Progress Committee, members discussed the problem. Everyone contributed to the talk. Members kept calm. They encouraged each other to share opinions. Finally, through discussion, a number of good ideas came up and the problem was solved for the time being.

At the end of this chapter is a section on holding meetings. It contains more about group behaviour, including how groups make decisions (page 167). The way a group makes its decisions can either help solve conflicts or make them worse.

The value of group education

Using the group approach to educate people has a number of advantages. First it provides support and encouragement. Maintaining healthy behaviour is not always easy. In a group one can find the support and encouragement needed to promote and maintain healthy practices.

Secondly, it permits sharing of experience and skills. People learn from each other. A member may have tried a new idea and found it successful. Through that experience the person has gained skills that can be passed on to other group members.

Finally, working in groups makes it possible to pool the resources of all members. One family may not have enough money to dig a well, but a group of families together could contribute enough money for the purpose. Members of a group can give money, labour, or material to help their members in times of personal or family crisis, or to promote community health through projects such as improving sanitation.

In sum, because some problems are difficult to solve by individuals alone, a group approach to health education is important.

We will now examine what steps need to be taken before we can plan health education activities with different kinds of group.

Education with informal gatherings

The first thing when dealing with an informal group is to find out what the common interests and needs of its members may be. Women who visit a market, for example, are concerned about good quality food at reasonable prices. Health education with informal groups should be based on common interests, whatever these may be. A topic of general interest to the women visiting a market might be 'Preparing inexpensive but nutritious meals'.

As you often do not know who belongs to informal groups, you may have to find out their needs through indirect means such as clinic records. That is what was done in the sample programme described below.

Another concern in educating informal groups is that the members may not know each other very well. You will have to develop relationships and encourage participation. Try to make people in the group feel welcome. Point out their common interests and needs.

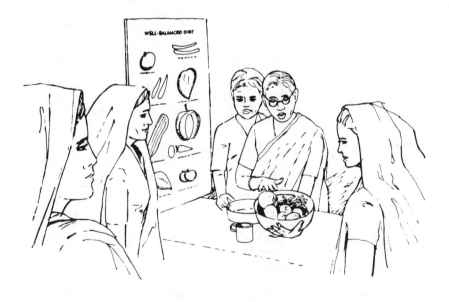

This health worker is carrying out health education for an informal gathering of women at the clinic. The health worker can use a variety of educational methods and aids in the programme—posters, demonstrations, story-telling, proverbs, etc.

115

A sample educational programme

Below is a sample educational programme prepared for mothers attending a preschool clinic. On the left side of the page are the activities and comments of the health worker who is presenting the programme. On the right side, reasons for these activities are listed. We assume the health worker has prepared all the materials that he or she will use well in advance of the presentation.

Sample educational programme prepared for mothers attending a preschool clinic

Topic: Treatment of diarrhoea at home	The topic should relate to the interests and needs of the target group. Clinic records may show that diarrhoea is a common problem. The topic is also a simple one. This makes learning easier.
Time: Early, before the health workers start to see patients	This is a time when people will be alert. There will be less disturbance. More people will be present.
Length: Planned for 20–30 minutes	The time is short, to prevent boredom. If the presentation lasts too long, mothers will become anxious about missing their turn with the health worker.
Format: Varied	Using a mixture of educational methods, like story-telling and demonstration, will make the programme more interesting. Also you can *repeat* the same ideas in different ways. This will ensure that people understand the ideas and remember them.

Opening comments by health worker

'Good morning. We hope that all your families are well'.	Opening comments establish a good relationship and friendly atmosphere. If people feel welcome they will be more willing to participate and share their ideas.

Using a poster

'Today we want to discuss a problem that many children have.'

Using a simple, one-idea poster helps to make points clear.

Health worker holds up a poster or photo of a child passing watery stools.

'What is happening in this picture?'

Asking questions encourages involvement and makes people think.

Mothers might say:
- the child is sick;
- the child is passing stools;
- the child has diarrhoea.

From the mothers' comments, you will know if the poster communicates the idea well.

'Thank you for your comments. Yes, the child is sick. She has diarrhoea.'

Praising ideas from the group encourages people to continue participating and learning.

'What we mean by diarrhoea is that the child is passing three or more loose, watery stools in one day. Is this what you mean by diarrhoea in your language?'

Mothers answer and explain.

Make sure communication is clear and that everyone understands what is meant by diarrhoea.
Consider local culture and the use of local words to communicate ideas.

'Have any of your children ever had diarrhoea before?'

Make sure that the topic relates to the needs and interests of the group.

Many mothers nod their heads and raise their hands.

Create a common bond of interest between group members.

'Yes, we all share this problem. Today we will work together to find out how to deal with diarrhoea when it happens to our children.'

Let mothers know they can participate in solving their own problems.

'Does anyone know what a mother can do when her child gets diarrhoea?'
Mothers may suggest:
- bring the child to the clinic;
- give the child herbal drinks;
- make the child rest;
- call grandmother for help.

Gather information on mothers' knowledge, beliefs, and experiences. Find possible solutions to the problem. Encourage participation in coming to understand the problem.

'Thank you for those ideas. It is true that a child with diarrhoea

By making use of ideas from members of the group, thereby

needs things to drink. She needs food and rest too. If the problem does not stop quickly, you should come to the clinic. Let's remember these ideas, and come back to them in a few minutes.

involving them in solving their problems, you will show that you respect and value people's views.

Using a story

'Now I want to tell you a story about two women I know whose children had diarrhoea.

Mrs Akpan and Mrs Oke are neighbours. Mrs Akpan is a seamstress, and Mrs Oke is a food-seller. Mrs Akpan's daughter, Grace, and Mrs Oke's daughter, Bisi, always play together'.

A story is a simple educational device that will create interest and make people think. Remember, do not use real names. It is good to use several devices. So far, a poster and a story have been used. The types of device used should:

- be familiar to the people;
- be easy to get or make;
- encourage participation.

'Last week when the two girls were playing, they picked up some fruit off the ground and ate it directly. Soon both girls had diarrhoea. When Mrs Akpan saw that Grace was passing watery stools, she became worried. She said "My daughter is losing so much water in her stools I had better give her things to drink and eat to replace what has been lost"'

'So Mrs Akpan gave Grace fruit juices, soup, clean water, and other things to drink. She fed Grace on soft foods such as porridge and bananas. Soon the diarrhoea was reduced'.

Mention locally available drinks and foods. Rice water and coconut water are other examples of suitable drinks. Pineapples and citrus fruits can be eaten.

'The next day, Mrs Akpan took Grace to the clinic. The health worker examined the girl. The health worker told Mrs Akpan that Grace seemed fine now, and that she should continue to drink juices, just as she had been doing. If the diarrhoea should trouble her again on the following day, she should come back to the clinic'.

Praise and encourage healthy behaviour.

'On the way out of the clinic, Mrs Akpan saw Mrs Oke rushing up carrying Bisi in her arms. Mrs Akpan ran over to see if she could help. She asked "What has happened?"
Mrs Oke said "Yesterday Bisi started having diarrhoea. I wanted to do something for her, but the old people in the house said I should leave her alone. They said that since too much was coming out, I should not put more food or drink in Bisi. I did what they said, but the diarrhoea never stopped. Now look, Bisi is all dried up and weak "'.

'Bisi was so dry and weak, she could not swallow. The health worker had to use a needle to put a special type of water into Bisi.' (The health worker now holds up a sample drip for the mothers to see.) 'Bisi stayed at the clinic for a couple of days. Now we are thankful that both Bisi and Grace are well and playing together again.'

To make the idea of the drip clear it is useful to demonstrate it. Emphasize that it would not have been required, if the mother had practised first aid with fluids available in the home.

Discussion of the story
'Let's discuss this story. What can we learn from it?'

Discussion of a story helps people think carefully about what they have heard. They can see the point of the story more clearly.

Mothers might say:
- children with diarrhoea need water;
- we should help our children quickly;
- children should not eat fruit that has fallen on the ground.

It will mean more to people if they can come to see a point by themselves. The ideas discussed will then have more value.

'Why did Bisi become so dry and weak?'
'What should Mrs Oke do if Bisi has diarrhoea again?'
'How can Mrs Oke explain these things to the old people at home?'

Other questions can be asked to encourage the mothers to think. Give several people a chance to answer after each question.

'So from this story we have learned that a child with frequent stools is losing a lot of water. We must do something quickly to replace that water. Remember how, in the dry season when there is no rain, the fruit of the orange tree becomes withered and tasteless. Oranges need rain and our children need water so that they will not wither away'.

Summarize the point of the story to help people remember.

Give a simple example to make the point more clear.

'Mrs Akpan acted quickly. It is most important for a mother to check if her child is becoming dry. Here are some signs to look for:

- three or more loose stools passed in a day;
- thirst more than normal;
- small amount of dark urine passed;
- eyes sunken;
- mouth and tongue dry;
- breathing faster than normal;
- when pinched, skin smooths out more slowly than usual.

If you see any of these signs when your child is having diarrhoea, bring the child to the health worker right away.'

Knowing limitations is important. Emphasize tasks that the mother can perform herself, and identify problems that require the assistance of health workers.

Active participation
The health worker then asks one mother to come forward with her child. Together they examine the child—looking at eyes, mouth, listening to breathing, and observing what happens to the skin after it is pinched.

It is important to ask the mother to try this observation of the child for herself. It will help her to learn.

'Now would all of you examine your children. Pinch their skin and see how fast it returns to normal.'

The health worker walks around and observes the mothers examining their own children.

All the mothers can then practise the skills learnt, while the health worker watches to see that they do so correctly.

'Could someone remind us of the things a mother should look for to see if her child is becoming dry?'	Repetition and questions help memory.
After receiving and praising correct answers, the health worker could ask 'What must we do if we see any of these signs in our children?'	When people give good answers and comments, thank them for their ideas and ask other people if they agree or have more comments.
The health worker thanks each mother who gives an answer, then says 'Please tell me some of the fluids and drinks you could give your child if he or she gets diarrhoea.'	
Some mothers answer 'milk' or 'spicy soups'. These are not appropriate, and the health worker should explain why, without criticizing the mothers who spoke.	If there are incorrect answers, other opinions can be asked for until someone gets the right idea.
'Now please say what foods a child with diarrhoea could eat.' Any suggestions of foods that may be rough on the child's stomach— whole grain foods or beans—would be politely discouraged.	Encourage mothers to contribute to finding solutions.
Demonstration 'Remember that Mrs Akpan gave Grace fruit juices and soup. These have water and other things that give the child strength and energy. I will show you a simple drink you can mix for your children that will give them water, strength, and energy when they have diarrhoea'.	Demonstration is useful for teaching skills. Just talking is not enough. The emphasis is on self-help. That is the educational objective. An explanation is given before the demonstration, so that the audience will know what is being done and why.
'You need: ● several cups ● boiled water (cooled) ● sugar ● table salt ● oranges, if available, for taste'.	If possible, use local materials that people recognize and can get easily. Provide enough of the materials to give everyone a chance to practise the skill.
'Give the child this drink each time he or she passes watery stools. Now watch while I mix the drink:	Explanations are also given at each step of the demonstration to make sure that people understand.

'First I am filling a clean cup with clean, boiled water. If the water is not clean, the diarrhoea may get worse.
'Second, I am adding a four-finger scoop of sugar'.

The correct size of cup or mug (about one-third of a litre) should be shown and explanations given.

The formula for mixing salt-sugar solution varies from country to country. Find out what is the accepted mixture in the area.

'Third, I am adding a pinch of salt; put three fingers together to take one pinch of salt. Do not add more'.
'Fourth, if I have an orange, I squeeze its juice into the drink to make it taste better'.
'Finally, I stir the drink so that no salt and sugar are left in the bottom of the cup. Now get the child to drink it slowly.'

The health worker should drink the mixture. This will show people that the drink is not bad.

'If a child drinks one cup of this each time he or she passes watery stools, the child will not lose too much strength, and will be able to get better faster. Allow the child to drink as much as he or she wants. Do not force-feed.

Recalling the point of the demonstration helps people remember.

'Do you have any questions? Would you like me to repeat any of the steps?'

Asking for questions from the group will help clarify points and make sure they are understood.

'Now could one or two of you come up to this table and practise making this drink yourselves? While you are mixing the drink, please tell us what you are doing'.

Practice is needed in order to learn a new skill.

'Would the others kindly give suggestions?'

Observation is needed to make sure that people are practising the skill correctly.

The mothers will taste the drink after they have made it. 'How does this drink taste? Could some more people come up and try to mix the drink?'

It is important that as many people as possible can practice the procedure. This will 'test' whether they have learned the new skill.

'This new skill you have learned today will help you when your children are sick. You should know, though, that many diseases can cause diarrhoea. Many times if you give this drink each time the child passes watery stools, the diarrhoea will stop after one day. If it does not you should bring the child to the health worker who will give you medicines to cure the disease.

When teaching a skill, it is important to let people know the limitations of the method. Here, the mothers are being taught to control simple diarrhoea, not how to cure disease. Just as community health workers are taught to refer some problems to health staff with more training, these mothers are being taught to refer certain problems to community health workers.

Concluding

'Before we close for today, do you have any questions about what we have seen and discussed?'

Make sure people are clear in their own minds about what they have experienced.

'Remember this picture?' (hold up the poster used at the beginning).' What should the mother of this child do?'

Wait for answers.

It is good to review the topic with a visual aid, because this will help people see the problem more clearly.

'Could someone remind us how to mix the special drink for children who have diarrhoea?

By asking questions, you are actually evaluating what people have learned.

'How often do we give this drink? 'What should we do if the diarrhoea does not stop after one day?'

If you have organized a good programme, the audience will have learned much and will be able to answer your questions.

When mothers give correct answers, say 'Thank you. That's right. You will be a great help to your child.' If the answers are not correct, say, 'Do the rest of you agree? What other suggestions are there?'

Praise correct answers to help people remember and value what they have learned. Do not embarrass people who give wrong answers.

'What other things should the child eat and drink in your opinion?'

Search around for other opinions until you find the right one.

Using a song

'Let us close with a song. Here is how it goes: 'A healthy child needs water to keep from getting sick; the ill child too needs water to make him get well quick.'

In many cultures, a song will help a meeting end on a happy note. It will give the audience a simple idea to remember.

'Now will everyone sing along? Can some of you think of more words for this song?' Repeat the song several times.	Everyone can participate in the singing and thereby have a feeling of belonging to the group.
'Thank you all very much for coming today. Now that you have learned these skills, your children should be much safer and healthier'.	It is important to ensure good relations right to the end. This will help people appreciate what they have just experienced and they will be glad to come back again.
'Remember the proverb 'Where there is water, there is life'.	The proverb should be part of the local culture and familiar to the people. It will show how the new ideas and skills taught are relevant to local values.
'Give my regards to your families. I hope all will be well until our next meeting. Good bye.'	

Meeting individual needs

When you educate people in a group setting like the one we have just described, you cannot always meet the needs of each individual. If you encourage participation, as in the example above, many people can take part. But you may not have time to deal with each person's needs and questions.

For example, one mother in the group may have grandparents living in the house. They may believe very strongly that a child with diarrhoea should not eat or drink anything. This mother may be afraid to tell the grandparents what she has learned. She will not be able to make use of her new skill until there is a chance for some individual counselling or a home visit from you.

Be sure to tell people in the group that they are welcome to meet you individually after the programme or at other times. If they have special problems or concerns, they can tell you about them privately. Then you can use the kinds of educational approach that work best with individuals to try to solve the problem. Counselling is one such approach; it was discussed in Chapter 4.

Education with formal groups

It is possible to plan a greater number and variety of educational programmes with formal groups. This is because formal groups have definite purposes and interests, specific leaders who can mobilize them, and commitment to meeting regularly and taking action. Since the members are known, it is possible to obtain greater cooperation from them in planning and carrying out a programme.

Identifying needs

Since we know who are the members of a formal group, we can ask them about their needs.

Suppose there is a fishermen's association in the community. A health worker meeting this group, may learn many of their needs. For example they may say:

'Two fishermen drowned last year so members want to learn life-saving and water safety skills.'

'When we are cleaning and preparing fish we often get cuts on our hands. When these become infected and sore, we cannot work very well.'

'New nets are needed. The old ones have been repaired too often. We want new nets made of strong material.'

'Much of the fish goes bad before it reaches the city for sale. We want better storage and transport facilities.'

'We want to learn to read and write so that no-one will cheat us when we go to town to sell fish and buy supplies.'

'We have a lot of problems with earaches and infections.'

Educational programmes could be planned with a fishermen's association, including courses on water safety skills, discussions on resources for economic development, and meetings on general health promotion in the community.

Attending meetings of a formal group

You cannot be a member of every group in your community. Therefore, when you attend a meeting of a community group, you are often an outsider. Before a group will cooperate with you on health and educational programmes, its members must know and trust you.

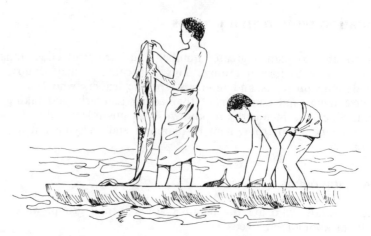

These men are members of a fishermen's association.

Before you meet with a group, it is best to see the leaders.
Explain what skills you have to offer. Find out if these would be
of any benefit to the group. If the skills can help the group solve
some of its problems, the leaders may invite you to a meeting to
talk to the whole group. They may also tell you that they will
report to their group what you have said. After the group has
discussed your ideas, the leaders will contact you. Of course it
would be nicer if you could explain your ideas directly to the
group, but never go to a group meeting unless you are invited.
Continue to show interest in the group, and in time the leaders
may trust you enough to invite you to a meeting (if that is
allowed by the group's rules).

When you attend a meeting, always show respect to the people in
the group. The leaders will often give you a set time at which to
speak. You should present your ideas clearly and simply. Do not
waste the group's time. Do not be surprised if, after the group
has finished discussing your ideas, you are asked to leave. The
group may have private business that it does not want to discuss
in front of a stranger.

If you stay through a whole meeting, do not make comments on
other items on the group's agenda, unless the leaders specifically
ask for your opinion. Once the members of the group get to
know you and see that you respect them, they may begin asking
for your opinions more often.

When you are presenting ideas to a group, it is important to
encourage participation in discussion. You will find useful
suggestions on ways to do this on page 130.

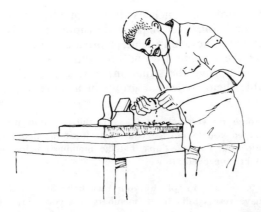

Carpenters are an example of a group of people with special needs and interests. Educational programmes can be planned with a carpenters' association or guild to help the members learn safe work practices.

Planning programmes

A formal group will be able to plan its own programmes and projects to solve its problems. A health worker could guide them in setting priorities, finding resources, and learning the skills needed.

During group meetings a health worker can present simple educational programmes like the one given on pages 116–124. More often the health worker will encourage the group to use meeting times to plan and carry out self-help projects, or to receive training in self-help skills.

Look at these sections of the book for ideas: Chapter 6, pages 191–193, on planning projects; this chapter, pages 158–159, on training; this chapter, pages 163–169, on holding meetings.

Helping a group to be successful

Once you have spent some time with a group, you will see whether the members are behaving in a way that will promote success or failure. If you have also been able to build a good relationship so that the members of the group trust you, you can try to help them improve their behaviour towards each other. If the members behave like those in the Unity Committee (pages 111–112), they will not be able to achieve any of their goals.

If you observe problems, such as disagreements, or uncooperative members, or confusion over making decisions in formal groups, you can meet with the group leaders privately. Find out what they think are the reasons for the difficulties. What have they done to try to improve the situation? You can teach them skills that will enable them to lead a group in a more successful way.

> To which groups do you belong? Can you think of how those groups have encouraged you to change your behaviour? In what ways do the members help you? Do you think that the members' behaviour in the group could be improved? How?
>
> Do you try to set an example by your own behaviour in the group? Do you behave respectfully to all members? Do you allow others to speak? Do you encourage others to express their views? Do you thank people for their contributions?

Discussion groups

From time immemorial people have come together spontaneously to learn from each other's experience and to discuss things. This interaction between people who have different views enables each of them to have a wider view of a problem. This is always very helpful.

Health education has been quick to recognize that groups provide an ideal set-up for learning in a way that leads to change and action.

Purpose

Discussion in a group allows people to say what is on their minds. They can talk about their problems. They can ask for help and suggestions from other members of the group. The group provides encouragement and support for people when they are trying to solve a problem and change their behaviour. Group support is important in helping people take decisions.

Size of group

Small groups are best for this type of sharing. Firstly because many of the problems people need to solve are personal and sensitive. They would not want to talk about their problems in front of a large group. Secondly, it is important that every member should have a chance to talk. Five people would be a good number. With more than ten, not everyone will have a chance to speak when he or she wants to.

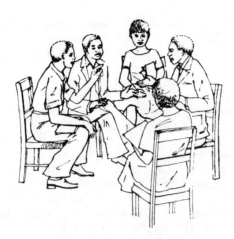

Five is a good number for a discussion group. People will be able to get to know and trust each other. Everyone will have a chance to participate in discussing the problems they share.

Planning a discussion

Common needs and interests
A discussion group can be formed around people with similar interests. Here are some examples:

- Parents of handicapped children.

- Women with problem pregnancies.

- Teenagers with worries about sexual matters.

- Patients suffering from a long-term disease such as diabetes.

Getting a group together
Talk to people individually to see if they would like to come together in a group to share their problems, find out how others cope, seek help, and in turn assist others.

Where to hold a discussion
Hold the discussion in a place that is comfortable and offers privacy. This will help people to talk more freely.

Holding a discussion

Build up relationships
Help people in the group to get to know each other. If they are from the same village or neighbourhood, they probably know each

129

other already. But do not assume that they know each other well. Allow time for each person to introduce himself or herself. People will feel more comfortable sharing their ideas in a group if they know each other.

Encourage others
You should encourage the people in the group to talk. You should not do a lot of talking yourself.

Begin with general knowledge
Discussion groups may meet several times. Therefore it is not necessary to ask people to talk about their problems and worries straight away. A good way to start might be to ask the group what general knowledge they have of the problem, illness, or worries facing them. Group members will begin to ask questions as they seek more knowledge.

Use questions to encourage sharing
Later, as the discussion gets going, you can ask questions like these:

* Have you ever asked for help with your problem? Who did you ask?

* Are any of you having difficulties in following advice given by health workers?

* Would some of you share the experiences you had in trying to overcome these difficulties?

Several people will raise issues. Do not try to answer them all yourself. First ask if other people in the group have ideas or suggestions.

Encourage participation
Watch carefully. If some members are being quiet, you might turn to them politely and ask, "Could you tell us your views on this issue?" If they do not join in after a few suggestions like that, do not force them to talk. Wait until the end of the meeting and then talk to them privately. Find out their reasons for being quiet. Once you know the reasons, maybe you can do something at the next meeting to improve the situation.

Of course some people may talk too much. Again you need to be polite. You might break in and say "That is an interesting idea. Let us hear what some of the others feel about it." If this does not work, see the person after the meeting. Explain the need for everyone to have a chance to talk.

Time

The time allowed for discussion depends on how much time members have. People have work, family, and other responsibilities. You yourself have other duties.

First ask members to set a time of day and week that is convenient for them. One to two hours would probably be the longest time you would want for discussion. Even if people do not have other things to do, they will get tired and bored if the discussion goes on for too long.

Check for satisfaction

Before a meeting ends, ask members if they are happy with the progress of the group. Do they think that they are learning? Do they think the group should continue? Are there any changes they want to make—in the time, the place, or the topics being discussed?

Self-help groups

Life is not easy for people who have special problems such as a long-term disease or a handicap. They need support and encouragement from family, friends, and the community, as well as from health workers. With support they can learn and practise the skills needed to make their lives better.

Purpose

People who suffer from the same problem can also give support to each other. For example, a person who has been blind for many years has had a lot of experience in trying to cope with life. He or she can give encouragement and suggestions to somebody who has recently become blind.

Group discussion is an educational method that can provide support for a small number of people. Larger numbers can be organized into a formal group or club (see Chapter 6, pages 177–180). Members of a club are in a better position to get resources than individuals acting alone.

A case study

This case study describes how one community nurse organized a club for people suffering from diabetes.

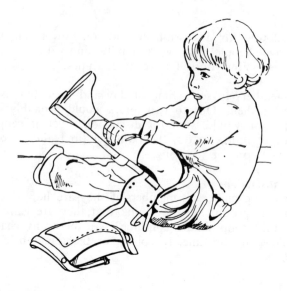

Parents of handicapped children can form a club or self-help group.

Identifying needs

The setting is a community hospital. There, one of the nurses, Sister Li, discovered that diabetic patients were having trouble following the recommended treatment. She observed that one quarter of the diabetic patients came to the clinic daily for urine-testing and insulin injections. They were unable to perform these by themselves. She also observed that at least five or six diabetic patients were often in hospital because they had not been taking good care of themselves. Clinic records revealed that over half of the diabetic patients did not keep the monthly appointment at which the physician would have reviewed their progress.

To shed more light on the problem, discussions were organized with a group of patients at the clinic. They indicated a number of reasons for their failure to keep monthly appointments: distance of the clinic from their houses, demands at work, long waits at the clinic, lack of transport, responsibilities at home, poor relationship with health workers, lack of understanding of the purpose of clinic appointments, and preference for traditional medicine.

The patients who did not test their own urine or give themselves insulin injections gave the following reasons for not doing so: they were afraid, they could not afford supplies, they were never taught the necessary skills, they lacked support at home, they believed that health workers did these things better, or they were embarrassed when people saw them testing urine or giving themselves injections.

Individual interviews with patients on admission showed that they had further problems: lack of understanding of self-care methods, difficulty avoiding foods they should not eat, the fact that people at home did not believe they were really sick, the belief that disease is caused by evil people casting spells, the feeling that they were causing trouble to people at home by requiring specially prepared meals, and the desire to be with friends who eat and drink normally.

Interviews during home visits confirmed that many of the husbands or wives, parents, and other relatives of the diabetic patients did not understand the disease and saw the patient's requirements as a burden or shame on the family.

With all this information, it was possible to see what kind of educational activities were needed to overcome the various problems noted.

An exploratory meeting

After she had found out about these problems, the nurse asked the patients and the hospital staff if they were interested in doing something to improve the situation. All were interested, so a meeting was held with several patients, three nurses, and one physician. Sister Li told the group that she had heard about diabetic patients in another town organizing themselves into a club for self-help.

The diabetic patients and the staff asked many questions about the club idea. Sister Li explained that the club would be run by the patients themselves. They could ask to have educational programmes and also teach each other self-help skills and provide support and encouragement. Staff members could give guidance to the club members. Everyone liked the idea of a club, so the group agreed to become the planning committee for a club for diabetics.

Gaining interest

Members of the planning committee held talks and discussions with other patients on clinic days. Individual patients were counselled and home visits were made.

A date was set for the first meeting. The local newspaper was contacted and asked to report on the event. Important people from the Ministry of Health and other agencies were invited. The meeting-hall was prepared with displays and posters. Seventy-five diabetic patients attended and joined in founding the club. They elected their leaders and began planning activities.

Developing programmes

It was decided that the club should meet once a month to conduct its official business. It was agreed to meet at a local school in the evening so that everyone would be able to attend, even the health workers.

Then the members decided that it would be necessary to organize an educational programme. A series of training sessions lasting for a period of two months were planned for each Wednesday, just before the regular clinic time. Patients would learn about their diet, urine-testing, how to give themselves injections, and other self-help skills.

133

Experienced patients and the health staff volunteered to be trainers. They also agreed to give individual counselling to patients in need. A counselling session would be held for all new diabetic patients to help them understand their disease and the necessary changes in their behaviour. Patients who were having trouble conforming to the advice of the doctor would also be counselled.

Club members and health staff also decided that home visits would be necessary to encourage the families of patients to provide the support needed at home.

Evaluation

After two months, the club discussed its progress at one of its meetings. It seemed that all but two patients were able to test their own urine and give themselves injections. Almost all patients were attending their regular monthly clinic appointment. At that time, only one patient was in hospital. Through self-help efforts, the diabetic patients were able to change their behaviour and improve their health.

Since this is a case study, you should think about it carefully. Do you agree with what the health staff and patients did? Could they have done anything differently or better? Would this type of club work in your community? What types of self-help clubs could be formed? What would have to be done differently for these clubs to succeed in your community? What could be done in the same way?

What were some of the ways by which the nurse collected information to be sure that there was a real need for and interest in the club? What methods did she use to encourage participation? What other educational activities might the club organize? What can the club members learn from their evaluation?

The school classroom

The school provides a good centre for health education. There, one will find groups of students and teachers. Teachers are resource people who can play an important role in primary health care and health education. Parents sometimes come to school to learn about their children's progress and to participate in meetings with teachers.

Teaching children about health

Children need to have adequate knowledge and skills and to develop the attitudes and values that will improve their health.

They need to be able to prevent the common problems that occur in their own community. They also need to know what to do if they should fall sick. Children should not only be given information. They need to acquire practical self-help skills.

Health education can fit in with many other subjects. In science classes, children often learn about insects and plants. They can be taught about insects that carry disease and what to do to prevent such disease. They can also learn about how to grow plants, and which plants are good for food.

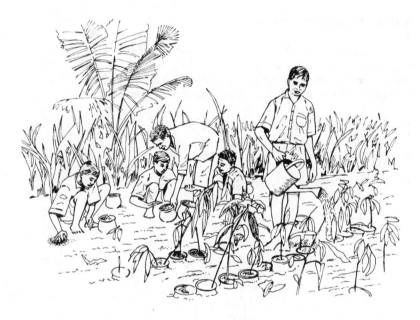

A garden can be a good project for a school class or a community club. The rest of the community can also learn new ideas and skills from a successful garden.

In language classes, children can read stories and act plays that have a health theme. When children learn spelling, they can be taught to spell words connected with health and illness.

During history classes, they can learn about famous people who discovered solutions to many of the world's serious health problems. They can also learn how health and disease have been connected with the progress and decline of nations and empires.

During physical education, they can learn skills that will build up their stamina and keep their bodies strong and supple.

Since children are young and active, it is good to use methods that allow them to participate fully in learning. They will value knowledge and skills that they gain through their own efforts. Methods that would encourage participation include: letting children ask questions, clubs, demonstrations, role-playing, plays, projects, games, community surveys, and discussions in small groups.

Older children should be able to help teach the younger ones basic health skills.

A healthy school environment

It is difficult to teach a child the value of health if the school environment is not conducive to healthy behaviour and if there are no resources with which to practise health skills. Here are examples of the health resources needed at a school:

- A clean and regular water supply.

- Hand-washing facilities.

- Sanitary means of disposing of human wastes/refuse.

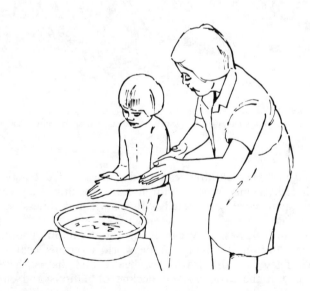

This teacher is demonstrating thorough hand-washing to a pupil. We cannot expect children to learn new health skills unless facilities such as clean water, soap, and a wash-bowl are available at the school.

- Well-lit and airy rooms.

- Playgrounds that are free from sharp and dangerous objects.

- First-aid supplies.

- Staff who are trained in hygiene and first-aid skills.

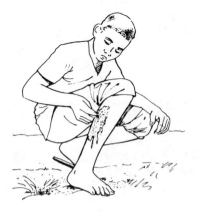

This schoolboy is rubbing sand on a wound that he got while playing football in the school yard. This could lead to infections such as tetanus. There are three possible reasons for the boy's behaviour: he believes that sand stops bleeding best; there are no first-aid supplies in the school; his friends want him to continue playing quickly. What kinds of health education programme could be organized in the school to solve such problems?

Teacher training

Although the Ministry of Education may say that certain health education topics should be taught in every school, this may not always be done. One reason is that the teachers may not have enough knowledge and skills to teach the subject. The school may not be lucky enough to have a staff member who has received training in health matters. Some teachers may have had such training many years ago, but may not know the latest ideas or may have forgotten what they knew.

In-service training can be organized for school-teachers. That means that teachers can receive training without having to leave their jobs. They may want to learn skills in first aid and the prevention of disease that are common in the community. See pages 158–160 for more ideas on organizing a training session.

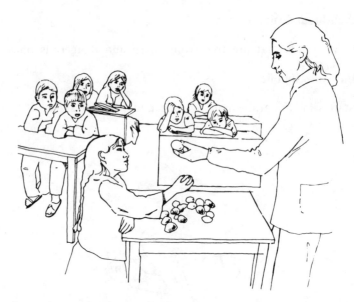

This teacher is using demonstration as an educational method. By showing children real-life objects — eggs and potatoes in this case — she can help them learn which foods help build strong bodies, and which give energy.

Parent and community participation

Ways should be found to encourage parents to play an active role in the health education of their children. In fact, parents are children's first teachers. Here are some ways in which parents can help with health and health education activities at school:

- Working together with pupils and teachers on self-help projects to provide the school with basic resources.

- Encouraging children to practise at home the health skills taught at school. For example children can learn to be observant about health problems, this awareness can easily be passed on to families.

- In certain cases, encouraging parents to come to the school and share their knowledge and skills—in other words, help teach. But this depends very much on the local culture.

It is often said that, since children are open to new ideas, they can carry these home to their parents. This is not as easy as it sounds. Many parents hold traditional beliefs that are very different from what is being taught at school. They may resent children who go against those beliefs. Also, parents may not have

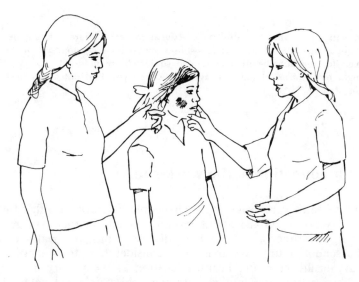

Schoolchildren can learn to be observant concerning health problems. This girl has discovered a discoloured spot on her classmate's cheek. Now the teacher may refer the girl with the spot to a health worker. Both girls are likely to go home and tell their parents about what has happened. In this way the health knowledge will be passed on.

the basic resources at home to allow the children to practise new health skills.

Home visits and family counselling may be useful in helping parents learn the new things that their children are learning. Meetings of parents with teachers are another way to provide health education for the parents.

Establishing links with other agencies and groups in the community is also necessary for a good school health programme. Health, community development, agriculture, social welfare, and other public and voluntary groups and agencies can provide valuable services to the school and its pupils.

Relationships

As a health worker, you are an outsider to the schools. You cannot just walk into a school and ask for the introduction of health education activities or for improvements in the teaching of health matters. You must meet with the authorities and staff. Build up trust and good relationships in the ways described in earlier parts of this book. Then you will be in a position to encourage the schools to make health education a valuable part of their programme.

> Do you know what the Ministry of Education says children should be taught about health? Do you know how much time is supposed to be given for teaching health and related subjects? Are different subjects taught to children at different ages? How can you find out about these things?

Health education at the work-site

Primary health care seeks to reach people wherever health care is needed. We have talked about reaching people in their villages and neighbourhoods, and we have discussed primary health care in the school setting. We must also consider how to organize primary health care and health education at the factory or work-site. This section does not go into the subject in great detail, but offers a few basic guidelines. You should apply the planning skills described in Chapter 3 to the work-sites in your own community.

What is a work-site?

People work in many places, including their own homes. Since this chapter is concerned with groups, this section discusses places of work where a group of people come together either to produce goods or to deliver a service. If, for example, the goods are clothing, the work-site could be as small as a tailor's shop staffed by the owner and two apprentices, or as large as a factory that employs over a hundred workers. The service could be a small eating-place where three or four people cook, serve, and clean up, or a large hotel serving hundreds of guests.

It is necessary to identify the different work-sites in your own town or neighbourhood. Also find out how many people work at each place and the different kinds of jobs they do.

Health and work

Health and work are closely related. People must work in order to feed and clothe themselves and protect themselves from illness. A person who is not healthy cannot work as well as someone who is. Then, too, the working environment can affect a person's health. Workers may be exposed to dangerous machines, hazardous chemicals, or stressful situations.

Health education at the work-site not only helps workers learn how to protect themselves from hazards in the working environment; it also teaches them how to take better care of their own personal health at work, at home, and elsewhere.

Planning work-site education

Obtaining approval

You cannot just walk into a factory or a business and begin health education. This would disturb the work going on. You first need to find out who is in charge at the work-site and gain their support and approval. At the same time you should find out when is the most convenient time for organizing educational programmes, where is the best place for holding programmes, and which different groups of workers may need education.

Seeking participation

Some large factories or service organizations are able to have their own health staff, but most work-sites are quite small and cannot afford a full-time health worker. It is important then for the workers to take part in selecting some of their own members to be trained in basic health promotion and first-aid skills. This will enable the workers to provide continuous primary health care for themselves through their own efforts.

Identifying needs

There are two main types of health needs that concern people at the work-site. First are those needs directly related to the work itself. Through observing, interviewing, and reviewing records (particularly if any are kept on injuries), one can identify the types of danger and stress to which the workers are exposed. Then there are the needs related to common problems that may affect a worker's personal health and ability to work. For example, malaria or alcohol consumption may be major reasons for absenteeism. Workers may be concerned about their cigarette-smoking habits. Health education at a work-site can focus on both occupational health hazards and personal health problems.

Training groups

Training is the organized teaching of new skills. It is most often given to groups of people, all of whom need to learn the same skills. Since training involves learning skills, there must be many opportunities for participants to practise their new skills, and to participate in the planning and running of the training programme to make sure it meets their needs. A planning committee made up of trainees and trainers is very useful.

Finding out training needs

We have already mentioned several groups in the community who could benefit from the training programmes you might organize:

- Community health workers need training in health care and health education skills.

- Teachers may need skills in health and health education.

- Various groups in the community may want to develop specific skills: for instance, pregnant mothers expecting their first babies may desire training in parenting and child-care skills, workers may want to train in first aid, and so on.

The following are some of the ways of discovering what kind of training people would like to receive:

- Talk to people in groups or during individual interviews. What skills do they want?

- Observe people at home and at work. Do they seem to be performing well, or is there room for improvement?

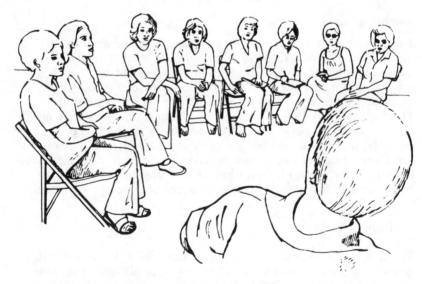

In group discussions and training sessions, it is important for everyone to participate. If the seats are arranged in a circle or a "U" shape, people can see each other and it is easier for them to discuss ideas and experiences.

- Look at the duties of the community health workers. Have they been properly taught how to carry out these duties?

- Think about the community. Are there special problems that require the community health workers to learn new skills?

- Read reports on, or review the progress of, programmes organized by your agency. Were the programmes successful? If not, do the programme managers feel that lack of skills among staff-members was a cause of failure? What do you think?

- Read magazines or newsletters put out by professional groups such as nurses and health inspectors. Also talk to your supervisors. What are some of the latest ideas in health care? What training is needed to practise the new skills?

Learning objectives

Training objectives

Training, like any other health education programme has an objective. The objective is the new behaviour that trainees will adopt by the end of the training programme. The behaviour in this case involves new skills. Examples of training objectives are:

- For a community health worker to be able to clean, treat, and bandage a small cut or wound.

- For a teacher to be able to demonstrate to pupils how to clean their teeth.

Health objectives

After community health workers, teachers, and other local workers have learned new skills, they should be able to provide better services. These should result in better health for the community. For example, training staff to carry out an immunization programme should result in the health objective of a marked reduction in the number of children who suffer from measles, polio, and other diseases, and the elimination of deaths from these diseases.

Involving people in setting the objectives

The people who are to receive the training should discuss their training needs and the educational objectives. They should agree on what they want to learn. In this way, people will be more interested in the training and will want to attend all the training sessions.

Training methods

A training programme should give people as much chance as possible to practise new skills. Health education methods that encourage participation and practice should therefore be used.

Audiovisual aids such as posters and projected material can give background information and knowledge. For training in the actual skills, techniques such as demonstrations, case studies, games, projects, and role-playing should be used. An example of an educational game can be found on pages 169–170. Descriptions of demonstrations, case studies, and role-playing are given below.

Demonstrations

Demonstrations are a pleasant way of sharing knowledge and skills. They involve a mixture of theoretical teaching and of practical work, which makes them lively.

Purpose

Demonstrations help people learn new skills.

Size of group

Demonstrations can be used with individuals and small training groups. If the group is too large, members will not get a chance to practise the skills or ask questions.

Planning the demonstration

Subject

Find out which skills the person or group needs to learn. You may be able to demonstrate the skill yourself. If not, find a person who knows the skill and can come and help you with the demonstration.

Materials

In a way, demonstrations are like displays with action. Some of the materials used for displays, such as models and real objects, can be used in a demonstration. Posters and photographs can also be shown.

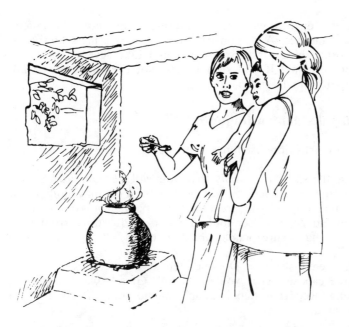

Demonstration is particularly useful when combined with a home visit. Skills will be easier to learn when the materials used are exactly the same as those with which the person normally works.

A demonstration must be realistic. Make sure that it fits in with the local culture. This means that you must use materials and objects that are familiar to the people who participate. You may be doing a nutrition demonstration. If people in the village use firewood and clay pots for cooking, use them too. Do not use unfamiliar things such as kerosene stoves and metal pots. Also use common food items. If you use strange or uncommon materials in your demonstration, people may not be able to practise the new skills at home.

Make a list of the materials you will need. Have them collected and ready on time. Have enough materials for everyone to use during practice.

Place

Plenty of space is needed for everyone to see the demonstration and to practise the skill.

Time

Choose a time that is convenient for everyone. Make sure that there is enough time for plenty of questions and practice. A simple demonstration of water-filtering would not take much more than 20 minutes. A demonstration to teach farmers how to build safe storage bins for their grain would take several hours. Allow for enough time. If you rush things, not everyone will be able to participate and learn.

Holding the demonstration

The demonstration itself has four steps.

Explain the ideas and skills that you will be demonstrating; photographs and pictures will help here. You may hold up some of the real objects you are using and pass them round for everyone to get a closer look. Encourage questions from the group to make sure people understand.

Do the demonstration. Do one step at a time, slowly. Make sure everyone can see what you are doing. Give explanations as you go along. Repeat a step if people do not understand it. Encourage plenty of questions.

Then ask one person to repeat the demonstration, and ask the group to comment as the person works.

Finally, give everyone a chance to practise. Move around the group and watch. Give suggestions for improvement. It is useful for people to work in pairs, so that they can have each other's suggestions and help. First, one person will practise the skill while the second watches and comments, then the second person will take a turn.

Planning for a series of demonstrations

Often it will take more than one meeting to teach people skills. Plan carefully. You may teach a few steps one day and then ask people to return the next day or the following week. Give people plenty of time so that they learn each step correctly.

You may be demonstrating to community health workers how to maintain and repair a bicycle. Think about how many steps or skills are involved. For example, they need to know how to fix a flat tyre. They must keep the chain greased and know how to put it back if it comes off. Plan one activity for each training session.

At the beginning of a new session, ask one of the group to repeat the demonstration of what was taught at the last session. This will help in checking if they have remembered.

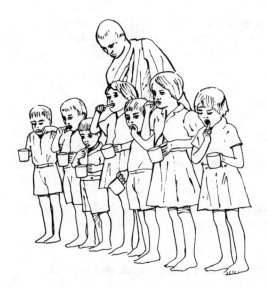

After demonstrating skills in oral hygiene to the schoolchildren, this health worker is giving them a chance to practise the skills. He is watching carefully to see that each child knows how to clean his or her mouth correctly.

Checking results

Check that everyone can practise the skill correctly before he or she leaves the demonstration place. You may be demonstrating how to mix a rehydration drink for children with diarrhoea. If a mother puts too much salt in the drink, she could harm her children. Before a mother leaves the demonstration place, make sure that she can show you that she will use the correct amount of salt.

Follow-up visits are useful in checking up on skills. In this way you will see if people can actually practise the skills on their own.

Case studies

Case studies are based on facts and present events as they really happened.

Purpose

Case studies help people learn how to solve problems. By reading or hearing about a case (or problem) in another group or community, people can begin to think how they themselves would have solved the problem. They will learn from the successes and mistakes of the people in the case study.

Size of group

Although you can discuss case studies with individuals, they are more interesting when read and discussed in a small group. That way more people can share ideas. This helps learning.

Case studies are useful with groups of schoolchildren, with community development committees, and during training sessions with, for example, community health workers.

Selecting and writing up a case study

First you must know what problems people want to solve. Let us say that you are working with a community development committee which has chosen to improve the village water supply. From your own experience, can you think of other villages that have tried to solve the same problem? Ask other health workers about their experiences in such projects, particularly if you have never been involved in one before.

Choose both successes and failures from among these experiences. Also choose experiences in communities with a culture similar to that of the community where you now work.

Write out these experiences to form the case study. If the village you are using for the study is near where you are working, change the name of the village and the people. They may become embarrassed if they learn that you are talking about them to people in neighbouring villages.

In the case study, describe each step that was taken to solve the problem. How did people first notice the problem? What did they think caused it? Who participated in trying to solve the problem? What action did they plan to solve it? How did they carry out the action? Did things go smoothly or were there difficulties? What were the final results?

Try to write briefly. The case study should be no longer than about two handwritten pages. If it is too long, people may not remember the details and may become confused when they discuss it. A sample case study is given on pages 150–151.

Using the case study

If the group can read, you may try to make a few extra copies of what you have written for them to share and read. If the group cannot read, you must read the case study to them. Read slowly. It is a good idea to repeat it to be sure that everyone has heard the main points.

After the case study has been read or heard, encourage group members to begin discussing it. You may ask a few opening questions. Do you agree with the solutions the people in the case study planned? Why do you think they succeeded (or failed)? Would the things they did work in our community? What should we do differently?

Encourage everyone to share opinions. Help the group reach some decisions about possible ways of solving the same problem in their own village or group.

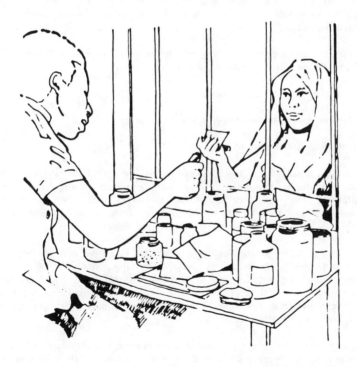

Community health workers are responsible for a small supply of essential drugs which enable them to provide treatment for simple health problems.

Sample case study
'Safe water for Amata Village'

The Iddo Community comprises a number of villages. In all of them, people suffer from guinea-worm infection, a waterborne disease. If people drink contaminated water, nine months or a year later they may find that a long, thick white worm has grown in their bodies. The worm usually grows in a part of the body that comes into contact with water (often the legs). The adult worm will cause an ulcer in the skin and push itself through so it can deposit its eggs in the water. This painful disease is responsible for many absences from work and school, and the ulcers can become infected with tetanus.

After discussing the problem with the staff at the local health centre, the residents of Iddo decided to organize a primary health care project to deal with guinea-worm and other local problems.

Word about the primary health care project was sent to every village in the Iddo area. Each village was asked to send at least one volunteer to the health centre to be trained as a community health worker.

The health centre staff drew up a training programme that took the problems mentioned by the community leaders into account, covering subjects like these:

● Clean water supply, including how to build wells, protected springs, and simple filtering, with emphasis on self-help;

● First aid for cuts and wounds.

● Treatment of simple problems like fever and diarrhoea.

● Health and nutrition of children.

Amata is a small village about 10 kilometres from the Iddo health centre. When the villagers heard the news about the primary health care programme, they were very happy. Out of the 75 people living in Amata, 40 were suffering from guinea-worm infection. They wanted someone to go to Iddo to learn how to rid the village of the disease.

When the chief of Amata heard the news, he asked his two brothers to come and discuss the idea. They decided that the son of one of the brothers would be sent to Iddo for training. This son, Amos, had finished primary school several years earlier. The three men thought that the boy was bright and thus a suitable choice. They also thought that the training might help him in the future.

When the decision to send Amos was announced in the village, people were not happy. Some had wanted to send members of their own families. They also thought that the boy was too young and might eventually run away to the city. He would be of no use to them then. A few people voiced their opposition, but the chief's mind was set. His nephew was sent for the training.

When Amos returned, the first thing he did was to call a meeting of the village elders. He said that the community should build a small hut or room for him next to his father's house. This room would be his 'clinic'.. It was the planting season and everyone was busy, but they agreed to do as Amos asked. They hoped that the clinic would help him work better.

Amos enjoyed treating sick people. He had been given a small supply of drugs in Iddo to use in his village. He had been told that he should charge a small amount of money for the drugs in order to be able to pay for replacements. Amos decided to charge more for the drugs and keep the extra money. The people did not complain at first, because they did not know how community health workers were acting in the other villages.

Amos tried to use up his drugs quickly. He would then go to Iddo to buy more. He would sometimes stay in Iddo, or even go to the city, for up to a week, enjoying himself with the extra money he had made from selling the drugs.

After a few months, the Amata people learned from friends what the community health workers in other villages were doing. Most of these workers had already started self-help efforts to dig wells and protect springs. None of them had asked their villages to build them a clinic. All were selling their drugs cheaply. The health workers in other villages were never away for a long time. When they went to collect new drug supplies, they usually returned on the same day.

The people of Amata were unhappy because they had not benefited from the primary health care programme.

Learning from the case study

A case study like this could be used with village leaders to help them learn how to select and use community health workers. It could be discussed with the community health workers themselves to help them learn how best to behave and work in their communities.

Here are some of the questions that might be discussed.

- What went wrong with the programme?

- What could the chief of Amata have done differently?

- What should those villagers who did not agree with his choice have done in the beginning?

- What is the best way of choosing a community health worker?

- What should be the qualifications of a community health worker?

- What should the people of Amata do now?

Then, on the basis of the ideas that come up during discussion, you could do a role-play. People could take the parts of the chief, his brothers, Amos, and several other villagers. One play could try to show how a good primary health care programme might have been organized in Amata. Another could try to show ways of improving the situation in which the people of Amata found themselves.

Role-playing

Role-playing consists of the acting-out of real-life situations and problems.

In a role-play, the player receives a description of the character he or she is to play. From the description, the player makes up the action and dialogue as the role-play progresses. The player tries to behave in the way that the character might behave when faced with a given situation or problem.

The participants simply behave in a natural way, so that their roles and the action develop as the play goes along.

In a role-play, people volunteer to play the parts. Other people watch carefully and may even offer suggestions to the players. Some of those watching might decide to join in the play.

After the play, players and watchers always discuss it and their reactions to it. Here, you have the important task of guiding the discussion. Ask the players questions like these: How did you feel? Are you happy with the way the situation you were acting worked out? Could you have done anything different to get better results? Then ask the audience to give their views. This discussion helps people to learn something from the play.

Purpose

By acting out a real-life situation, people can better understand the causes of their problems and the results of their own behaviour. Role-playing can help an individual explore ways of improving his or her relationships with other people, and of gaining other people's support in efforts to live more healthily.

Another purpose of role-playing is to give people experience in communication, planning, and decision-making. Finally, it helps people to reconsider attitudes and values. We learn about our own behaviour during a role-play. We can discover how our attitudes and values encourage cooperation and problem-solving or, how our attitudes and values create problems.

Group size

Role-playing is usually done with small groups. A role-play can be done with a health worker and one or two other people. Someone may come to a health worker in private. The health worker may ask the person to act out their own problem. The health worker would play the part of someone important in the other's life.

Time

A role-play should last about 20 minutes. If the action is lively and the audience is interested, allow the play to continue. But you should stop the play if (a) the players have solved the problem; or (b) if the players are getting confused and cannot solve the problem; or (c) if the audience looks bored.

Allow another 20–30 minutes for discussion. Discussion helps people focus on the important issues in the play. If the discussion is lively, allow it to continue longer. You may suggest a repeat of the play to try out the suggestions that have resulted from the discussion.

Other concerns

Role-playing works best when people know and trust each other. Before using role-playing with an individual, be sure you have established a good relationship with that person. If a group is involved, be sure that the members have already met a few times so that they know each other.

Role-playing involves some risk. Since we do not know the outcome, players are taking a chance when they act in a role-play. Do not ask people to take parts that might embarrass them. Some people may not be interested or may be very afraid to speak out in a group. Do not force such people to take part. Let them watch role-plays a few times to see if they become less timid or more interested.

A sample role-play

Mrs Debo is a community nurse. She has organized a mother's club in one village. The club meets once a month at the district health centre to discuss ideas about raising children, and to learn new skills. One day three of the mothers came to see Mrs Debo. They asked if the club could meet at the local primary school that month. They said that the school was closer to where most mothers lived. Mrs Debo saw from their eyes that there were probably other reasons for the change of place. She decided not to ask any questions at that moment and agreed to the change. When the club met at the school, they told Mrs Debo their problems. They said that the staff at the health centre were not nice to them. Sometimes the record clerks kept the mothers waiting a long time. If the mothers asked about their cards, the clerks would be rude and tell them to go home if they did not want to wait. The mothers claimed that the nurses yelled at them if their children were not gaining enough weight. The nurses only gave orders, they never explained anything. If a mother asked for an explanation, the nurse would say she was too busy. Finally, the staff at the dispensary also kept the mothers waiting. The dispensers would have drugs for their friends ready within five minutes, but many mothers would have to wait an hour. Then when they got the drugs, there would be only half the recommended dose. If they complained, they were told to buy the drugs elsewhere.

Now Mrs Debo knew why the mothers wanted to meet at the school. They were afraid of the health centre staff. They did not want to make their complaints where someone would overhear them.

Mrs Debo decided to use role-playing to help the mothers and herself learn more about the problem. She told the mothers what a role-play was and asked if they would like to try it. They all agreed they would. She started with the problems with the record clerks. The health centre had two clerks, so she asked two mothers to volunteer to play the clerks. Then she asked the rest of the mothers to play themselves. They moved some tables together and pretended to be in the records office. Then the play started.

1st mother: (walks up to clerks' office) I need my card, my child is very sick. He's been vomiting since yesterday.

1st clerk: If the child is so sick why didn't you bring him yesterday? Wait, I'll get the card (both clerks walk away).

2nd mother: (walks up, sees no-one at desk) Hey? Anyone here? My baby is sick, I need my card.

2nd clerk: (yells from back of office) Can't you people wait? We're looking for the other woman's card.

2nd mother: So it takes two grown men to find one small card?

1st clerk:	You can go home if you can't wait.
1st mother:	I've been waiting too long already. The government pays you a good salary. You should work for it. I wish my husband had a job that paid as much as that.
2nd clerk:	It's not my fault you married a poor man.
1st clerk:	(finally brings the card—for which a small piece of paper can be used) Here, take this (lets the card drop to the floor in front of the table).

The play continued like this for a while with a few more mothers coming up to get their cards. Their words were similar to those of the first two mothers. Then Mrs Debo stopped the play so that everyone could discuss what they saw. The discussion went like this:

Discussion of the role-play

Mrs Debo:	Would the mothers who acted the clerks tell us how it felt to be a clerk?
2nd clerk:	I was not too happy with the job. The second mother was not very polite. I did not feel like finding her card.
2nd mother:	Why should I be polite to those clerks? They are all younger than me. They are paid a good salary for doing their work.
Nurse:	Is it necessary to be polite only to older people?
3rd mother:	I was always taught by my mother to be polite to everyone. You never know where you will meet people in this life. It pays to be polite.
1st mother:	But shouldn't the clerks be polite to us first? Neither of them said good-morning or asked how our children were.
1st clerk:	I guess we were busy and forgot to greet you, but you did not have to insult us. Your attitude suggested we were stupid when we did not find the card quickly.
4th mother:	I think that all of you were insulting each other. I think we can behave better than that. If we wait for someone else to be polite first, we may have to wait a long time. We should make an effort to be friendly and polite. Maybe that will teach the clerks a lesson on how they should behave.
Mrs Debo:	What do you all think of this last comment?

The women nodded their heads in agreement; some of them said 'Yes. That's right.'

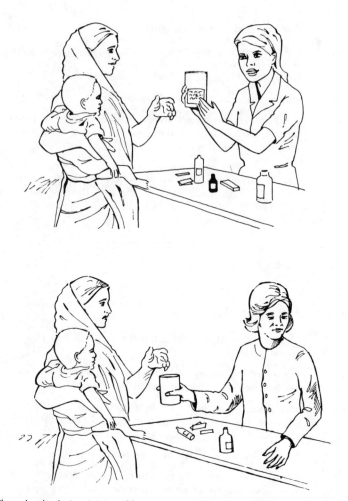

Through role-playing, it is possible to portray positive or negative types of behaviour and to show their impact. For instance, patients will be more likely to take their medicines properly if they receive a careful explanation (as in the top drawing) than if the drugs are handed to them casually (as in the bottom drawing).

As the discussion continued, the mothers agreed to try to be more polite to the clerks, even if the clerks did not say anything nice to them first.

They repeated the role-play with different volunteers. Everything went much better the second time when the mothers tried to be polite.

One issue still remained. The mothers said that the clerks started being rude some years ago. Because of this the mothers had become ruder themselves. They wished that someone would talk to the clerks about this problem. Mrs Debo agreed to see the clerks. They decided to wait until the next meeting before discussing the problems with the dispensers and nurses. If there was an improvement with the clerks, then they would try to solve the other problems.

Mrs Debo kept her promise and met the clerks. She did not tell them directly about the mothers' feelings. That might have made them angry. She simply talked to them about their jobs. Were they happy? What did they like about their jobs? What problems did they have?

The two clerks said that the job was not bad compared with other government jobs, but they had difficulty supporting their families on the small salary. They complained that many of the patients demanded too much. The clerks felt that the local people did not like them because they were from another district.

Mrs Debo found out a number of things that day. She knew that the mothers and the clerks did not understand each other very well. For example, the mothers felt that the clerks were rich because they worked for the government. The clerks felt that the mothers did not like them because they came from another district. Mrs Debo asked the clerks if they would like to try a role-play to learn how they could handle the patients better. They agreed. Mrs Debo pretended she was a mother. She behaved in the way the mothers had behaved in their role-play. Then she asked one of the clerks to pretend that he was a mother. After the play and discussion, the clerks came to understand the problem better. They realized that they could be more polite. They also realized that when a mother is worried about her sick child, she sometimes forgets to be polite.

When the mothers had their next meeting, they thanked Mrs Debo. They said that they had seen a big improvement in the clerks. One mother said that when she became friendly with them, she learned that one clerk was married to a relation of hers. She had since invited the clerk and his family to her house. The clerks also told Mrs Debo that they had seen a big improvement in the patients.

By using role-play, this community nurse had helped mothers and clerks change their attitudes and learn new skills for communicating with other people, thereby changing their behaviour.

Get together with some other health and community workers. Decide on a problem and make up a role-play. It does not necessarily have to be a personal problem of your own. It could be a problem in the village in general. Get volunteers to play the different parts. Practise several times to get the 'feel' of what a role-play should be. After practising with a group of people you know, try to use role-playing with a patient or a community group.

157

A group training session

Planning

Several important factors need to be kept in mind.

While you can certainly help people to acquire new skills, you may not know everything the participants want to learn. You may need to bring in resource people who have special skills to share with the others.

How long will it take for people to learn the new skills? Remember to allow enough time for everyone to practise. Some training programmes last a few days, others a week, a month, or longer. This depends on how much needs to be learned.

The time should be convenient for the trainees. Can they take time off work? Are they able to meet only once a week? Is daytime or evening better?

Find a meeting-place that is big enough to hold all the trainees. Make sure the place is comfortable and that eating and toilet facilities are available. Find a place that is easy for all trainees to reach. You may be able to use a local hall or school without charge.

Educational material such as posters, projectors, and photographs may be needed. Also trainers will need material with which to practise their new skills.

This should be obtained well in advance. Use educational material that you can make yourself, as far as possible. Try to plan training programmes using local materials and resources.

What about transport and housing? Are these needed for your particular training session? Find out if there are people who would be willing to transport and house your trainees.

If money is needed, contributions might come from the trainees or from various agencies. Money received for the programme must be carefully and accurately accounted for, so that one can see where it came from and how it was spent. Also note that people may be glad to contribute again in the future if they are thanked for their donations. In any case, you must express appreciation for the support you have received.

Running the training session

Pay attention to relationships by making sure that all the trainees and trainers know each other. In this way they will work better together.

Review the proposed objectives and activities with the trainees at the beginning of the session. This is a good idea even if you have involved them in the planning. Make sure that the plan is acceptable. Ask for suggestions for changes. If time and other resources allow, make the desired changes, but make sure first that everyone agrees to them.

In order to encourage participation, trainees should lead sessions, demonstrate skills, share their own ideas and experiences, and make suggestions for improving the programme as it goes along.

A training programme should be flexible. This means that the trainers should be willing to make changes at any time to make sure that the programme will be successful.

Evaluating the training

Evaluation occurs throughout the programme. The following questions will help you think about how you will evaluate the training.

- During the training sessions. Is the learning of skills and the availability of resources going as planned?

- At the end of the programme. Can all the trainees practise the skills they have been taught?

- After the programme. Are the trainees able to put their new skills to use in the community?

- Are there changes in the health behaviour of the people in the community?

Think of training programmes you have attended. Did they always have clear educational objectives? Did you always participate in setting out the training needs? Did the educational approach and the material used allow you plenty of experience with the new skills taught? What problems do you think the organizers may have had?

Which was the best training programme you ever attended? What made it so good? Which was the worst training programme you have been in? Why was it so bad? What could have been done to improve it?

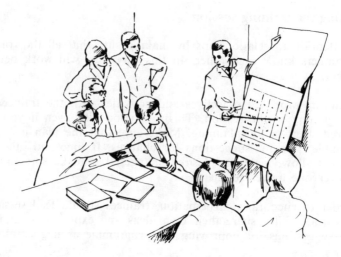

Training programmes should apply the very methods that health care workers are later expected to use with the community. Presenting the problem clearly, getting participants to discuss ideas and facts, and then getting them to propose realistic solutions—all this leads to involvement and action.

The health team

What is a team?

A team is a special type of group. Like other groups, the team has a purpose or goal. In a team each member has special skills or responsibilities. It is necessary for every member of the team to work together and to cooperate if the team is going to succeed in its tasks.

A football (soccer) team is an example. Each of the eleven players has responsibility for a particular part of the football field. If each team member does not handle his or her responsibility well, the team will probably score no goals. No one team member is more important than another.

It may be true that only one person kicks the ball into the goal, but if the other members of the team had not been doing their job, this one person would never have had the chance of scoring.

Members of the health team

The goal or purpose of the health team is to improve and maintain the health of the community it serves. In order to achieve that goal, the health team is made up of different members who have been trained in special skills. Think of the staff at your local health centre, dispensary, or clinic. There may be nurses, public health inspectors, health aides, records clerks, dispensers, midwives, medical assistants, and maintenance staff.

All of these people must work together to make sure that health care reaches people in the community.

Of course the physician is a member of the health team, but not every health centre or clinic will have a doctor present all the time. Many have doctors who visit once a week or once a month. Sick people who cannot be treated at a health centre are referred to the nearest hospital where the health team is much larger and may include doctors, nurses, midwives, laboratory technicians, X-ray technicians, and hospital aides.

The larger hospitals may also have dentists, physical therapists, pharmacists, health educators, administrators, and social workers.

Responsibilities of team members

Let us look at the example of a child health programme in a local health centre. The nursing staff examine both well and ill children to see how they are growing. They treat some sick children and refer others to the doctors. They provide preventive services such as immunization. The dispensers provide medicaments for sick children and keep a supply of vaccines for prevention.

The midwives try to see that healthy babies enter the world by providing antenatal care and a safe delivery. Then midwives follow the children up as they begin to grow. The records clerks maintain records in good order so that the history and progress of all the children can be seen easily.

The environment in which the children live must be healthy. Through home visits and community projects, the public health inspector works towards a healthy community environment. The maintenance staff at the centre or clinic guarantee that the place will be clean and welcoming.

These are just a few of the responsibilities of each team member. All are important for promoting child health. The situation will be similar in any health programme.

Team leadership and cooperation

Like formal groups, teams have leaders. The leaders, however, are not elected, neither do they inherit their positions. In fact the leaders may change from time to time depending on the project.

For the normal administrative work of the team, it is often the most senior or experienced member of the nursing or environmental health staff who organizes the team's activities at a health centre. When a doctor is present, she or he usually takes on that responsibility.

The leadership of a specific project will depend on what the project is about. If the project is mostly concerned with the health of pregnant women, the midwife or the nurse will naturally give leadership and direction to team efforts. Should the project deal with environmental hygiene, the sanitarian, health inspectors, or health superintendent will assume leadership.

What we have said so far about sharing responsibilities and cooperation belongs to the domain of the ideal. Teams do not always work so well together. While a football team practises together regularly, members of a health team sometimes tend to work on their own. It is sad when they do not share their experience and do not ask other team members for help.

Health education methods and skills can be used to encourage better team work. Each member should try to promote good relationships and communication among all team members. When there are projects to work on, ways should be found for everyone to participate and contribute their particular expertise.

Discussion groups and meetings (see the next section on conducting meetings) are useful tools for helping the team plan and evaluate programmes. It is. through regular meetings that progress can be evaluated, relationships can grow among members, and new problems can be identified and solved.

When the team does meet, observe the behaviour of the members, including yourself. Do they make for a healthy and successful group? Think about the Unity and Progress health committees we discussed on pages 111–113.

If a health team works in the same way as the Unity committee, it will never achieve its goal of improving community health. Health education skills can encourage mature group behaviour like that of the members of the Progress Committee.

Health education duties of team members

The health team is a place where members can work together to improve their health education skills. These skills can serve to improve the quality of the team-work. They should also be used when the team carries out any programme. During team meetings, members can decide who will be responsible for which types of health education.

In the child health programme, the nurses can arrange programmes for informal groups of mothers at the clinic. They can also give individual counselling to mothers and children with problems. The environmental health staff can organize community meetings and projects. The dispensers can educate patients about their drugs, so that they will be able to take them correctly.

Think of other educational activities that would be appropriate for each team member.

Suppose you are organizing health programmes for (a) the teenagers, (b) the elderly, and (c) the farmers in your community. What would be the responsibility of each health team member in each of these programmes? What would be the health education duties of each member? How should other community workers be involved in such programmes?[1]

Meetings

A common activity of most of the groups described in this chapter is the holding of meetings to discuss and solve problems. This section considers what is needed to conduct good meetings.

There are different kinds of meeting. Some involve general participation in the discussion and in taking decisions (committee meetings, board meetings, public meetings on an issue of concern to the community). Others, like the annual assembly of an association, use a few speakers who address a largely passive audience. In health education we are concerned with the first type of meeting.

---

[1] See also: MCMAHON, R. ET AL. On being in charge. A guide for middle-level management in primary health care, Geneva, World Health Organization, 1980, pp. 61–140.

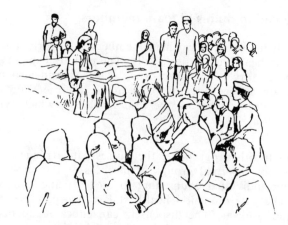

There are many types of meeting. A small group of community leaders can get together to discuss health problems and take decisions. Or a whole community can assemble to hear about a health problem and give their views on it. Each kind of meeting requires a different approach.

Purpose

Meetings are held to gather information, share ideas, take decisions, and make plans to solve problems. Meetings are different from group discussions. A group discussion is free and informal. Meetings tend to be held for a special reason and are more organized. They have, for example, appointed or elected leaders. Meetings are an important part of successful self-help projects.

Size of group

In meetings held by organizations and associations, 20 to 50 people may come together. Community leaders may have small meetings where 5 to 10 people take decisions about community needs. On the other hand, the whole community can come together in a meeting to learn about problems and express their views.

Planning a meeting

Need

It is important that the members of the organization or the community see the need for a meeting. Does the problem require a meeting, or can it be handled easily by one or two members?

The decision to hold a meeting should be made by the group members or community leaders themselves.

Time and place

Many organized groups have regular times and places for their meetings. The village heads may meet once a week at the Chief's house. The neighbourhood council may meet monthly in the community hall. The tailor's guild may meet every two months at a school or mosque.

Make use of regular meetings to solve problems and set out plans for action. If a special meeting is necessary, the leaders of the group should decide on a time and place that will be convenient for all.

Announcing the meeting

Each group or organization has a way of informing members about meetings. This may be by posters, town criers, or word of mouth. The group should make the announcement itself.

Word of mouth is often the best way to announce meetings in a village or small neighbourhood. The need for the meeting can be announced by the leader to the people he or she works closely with. These people then spread the word to others, who in turn tell others, and so on.

Announcements will spread more quickly and reliably if a system to facilitate communication is set up. In such a system, each member of the group has the responsibility of contacting certain other people. Here is how it might work:

The leader will contact four people to announce the meeting. Each of these people knows the names of four other people whom he or she will contact. These people in turn will contact others.

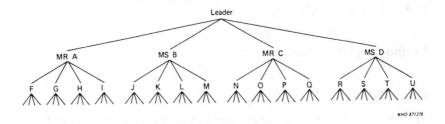

One way to do this is to look at the different sections of the village or neighbourhood. There should be someone in each section for the leader to contact first. If Mr A is away when the leader tries to contact him, Mr F could then fill in for Mr A.

Meetings should be announced several days in advance to give people time to prepare. But do not announce the meeting too far in advance or people may forget when it is.

Preparing an agenda

An agenda is a list of the topics or issues that will be discussed at a meeting. This should be planned carefully. People will lose interest if they come to a meeting where no one knows what is supposed to happen.

If the group already has leaders, see them some days before the meeting. Discuss the agenda. There may be issues remaining from the last meeting that must be discussed first. There may also be new topics to add. An agenda should not be too long. Ideally, it should include only one or two important topics. A long agenda means a long meeting. After one hour, people start to get tired. After two hours, they start to leave. If people leave before the work is finished, the group may not be able to solve its problems.

Also, a long agenda may force people to make quick decisions which they may regret later. When the agenda has been agreed upon, look at the topics listed. What information will the group need to be able to discuss the topics carefully? If the members of a farmers' cooperative want to meet to discuss ways of improving their crops, they will need information on types of fertilizer including their cost and effects. Some of the group leaders should volunteer to find out this information. You can guide them on where to look. Do not do it all by yourself. It is useful for people to learn how to find information and resources.

When the meeting is announced, also tell people briefly what will be on the agenda. This will help them prepare. Members can look for information themselves. They can begin to think of ideas to be put before the meeting.

Conducting the meeting

Leadership

Most organizations, associations, and councils have their own leaders. These are the people who should be in charge of the meeting. You will have already given them encouragement and suggestions during the planning of the agenda.

You should speak when the leaders request it and should occasionally give other comments. Be sure that the other members of the group have the opportunity to speak their minds fully.

Participation

Participation in the meeting depends on the culture of the community. In some places leaders do most of the talking. In others, every member speaks. Encourage the kind of participation that is acceptable to the people. You can add comments like the following to encourage more people to talk:

- 'It would be useful if we could hear more about this flooding problem from the people who live near the stream.'

- 'This problem of dog-bites worries us all. I am sure those members with small children must have some experience in this area that they can share with us.'

Make issues clear

Before the meeting can reach intelligent decisions, everyone must understand the problems and the suggested solutions. Comments like these can help:

- 'Is everyone clear about how much money this project will require?'

- 'Does anyone want us to explain again how these immunizations work?'

- 'Does everyone understand what will be the responsibility of the community and of the sponsoring agency in implementing this project?'

Reaching decisions

Here are four ways in which decisions can be made in meetings:

- The group as a whole discusses an issue. After some time the leader or another member may say 'I think that we all agree to take this action. Does everyone feel this way?' At this point anyone can object. If there are objections, then discussion continues until there is a final sense of agreement. This is called consensus decision-making.

- The leader listens carefully. When he or she senses that everyone is in agreement he or she announces a decision.

- An issue can be placed before the group and members can be asked to vote on it. Action is taken according to the majority vote, that is, action is taken on the idea that the largest number of people prefer.

- The leader alone may decide on what he or she thinks is best and announce that the decision stands for the whole group.

The first two methods are very similar. In both cases a decision is not taken until there is general agreement in the group. This may take longer than voting or than the leader deciding for the group, but it encourages participation. When everyone is in agreement, action is very likely to follow. It is a good idea to make a note of what is agreed at a meeting so that people do not forget.

Taking action

The purpose of a meeting is to decide on plans that will help solve a group or community problem. Look at Chapter 3 for ideas on planning. Simply put, the group must:

- Set objectives (desired results).

- Decide on strategies (ways to solve the problem).

- Find resources.

- Set a timetable for action.

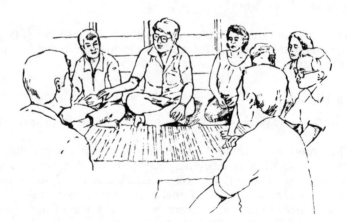

A group can reach decisions in various ways. In some groups the leader tends to decide. In others, the whole group has to come to a consensus or an agreement. When everyone agrees, action is much more likely to follow than when only one or a few people feel involved.

- Arrange for tasks to be carried out by individual members or small groups of members (committees).

- Meet regularly to review progress and make improvements or changes in the plan as necessary.

> Think about meetings you have attended. They might have been staff meetings in your agency, community meetings, or meetings of various organizations. Why did some meetings turn out successfully? Why did others have problems? What did the leaders do to make the meeting run smoothly? Did the leaders create any trouble? Why was that? In what different ways did the groups make decisions? What happened when people were not happy with decisions?

An educational game about decision-making

Here is a simple game you can use to help people learn about making decisions. No materials are needed. Twenty or more people are usually required. If there are fewer than fifteen people you will have to divide the group into two instead of three, keeping 'Group 1' and choosing either 'Group 2' or 'Group 3' (see below) as the other group.

Divide the group into three equal-sized smaller groups

Ask each group to select a leader. Explain to the groups that they must try to decide what is the most important problem in the community.

Meet separately with the leaders first

Tell the leader of Group 1 that he or she must encourage decision-making by consensus in that group. Explain carefully what consensus is. Tell the leader of Group 2 that he must force his group to agree with whatever decision he himself makes. Tell the leader of Group 3 to ask the people to vote on the different suggestions put forward.

Allow each group to meet

Make sure there is space for each group to meet separately so that they will not disturb each other.

Give plenty of time for the game

It may take some hours to reach a decision. You may have to ask the groups to report back the next day with their decisions.

Bring everyone back together

When the groups have reached their decisions, get a member from each group to explain how they reached their decision. Have various people say what they thought and felt. In Groups 2 and 3, you will probably find some people who are unhappy or angry because the group decision went against their views.

Ask the groups to report on what they have learned

Ask if they feel that what they have learned will improve the way they work together to make decisions in the future and if so, what sort of improvements they expect.

Chapter 6

Health education with communities

Enabling communities to gain the skills necessary for the safeguard and promotion of health is a major objective of health education.

Through community involvement, lay and professional people study health problems, pool their knowledge and experience, and develop ways and means of solving the problems. Our role is to help the community organize itself so that learning will take place and action will follow.

This chapter discusses:

- What a community represents (pages 172–173).

- When community health education is needed (pages 174–175).

- Getting opinion leaders involved (pages 175–176).

- The role of local organizations (pages 177–180).

- The community health committee (pages 180–183).

- Advisory and planning boards (pages 184–186).

- Intersectoral coordination groups (pages 186–187).

- Organizing a health campaign (pages 187–189).

- Special community events (pages 189–190).

- Mobilizing community resources for a project (pages 191–193).

- Developing a partnership with people (pages 193–194).

- The role of the community health worker (pages 195–196).

Linking together people from different sectors such as education, agriculture, industry, labour, town-planning, etc. to work out their own solutions to their problems – with the guidance of health and other community workers – is the surest way to health progress and development.

What is a community?

People who share common interests and have the feeling that they belong together form a community. In a community people usually share common values, a common history (or background), and accept certain forms of behaviour as normal for all community members. People belonging to a certain religion or having the same political beliefs could also be called a community.

A community, then, is not the same thing as an area of land. Community is people, not land — but community members will often be able to point out the boundaries of land that belongs to the community.

We can demonstrate this by taking the example of a small village. The houses and farms of the village may occupy 50 hectares of land. We cannot say, though, that the land with its houses and farms is the community. There are possibly sons and daughters who have moved away to larger towns and cities. They may have their own children and grandchildren there. Yet, they may still feel that they are members of their original village community. Another possibility is that the village land is occupied by groups of people from different backgrounds. In that case, the village may shelter two or more communities. Feeling part of a community is a feeling of belonging that people hold in their minds and hearts. A community cannot be identified simply by looking at the land or lines drawn on maps.

Identifying communities

Here is a case study that shows why it is necessary to identify clearly the communities with which we work.

> Mr Jola is a health assistant working in a small dispensary that serves ten villages. He would like to involve the people more in providing their own health care. He visits all the villages to see if they would be willing to have a volunteer trained in primary health care. He stops at the first house in each village and asks the people to take him to the village leaders. So far, all have agreed to participate in the programme and to send volunteers for training. Several months later, there is a cholera outbreak in the next district. Mr Jola meets with the volunteer community health workers to discuss what should be done to protect the people. After several suggestions are made, the community health workers go back to work out specific plans in their own villages.
>
> In a few weeks, the cholera has spread to Mr Jola's district. Fortunately, because of the advance planning, most villages were prepared. Few people

became sick and none died except in one village, Abedo. There, twenty people, all from the west side of the village, died of cholera. This seemed strange, so Mr Jola went to Abedo to investigate

On reaching Abedo, Mr Jola met the community health worker and asked to visit the section of the village where the people had died. Mr Jola talked to the families in that section and made an interesting discovery. These people said that they had originally come from a place about 50 kilometres away. Although they now lived in Abedo, they still had their own leaders, celebrations, and customs. They had never worked closely with the people who were native to Abedo, so they had not participated in any of the primary health care activities to prevent disease. Even though the map showed that these people lived in Abedo, they were really a separate community.

How could Mr Jola have avoided this problem in the beginning? What steps are needed to make sure that a community is correctly identified and involved?

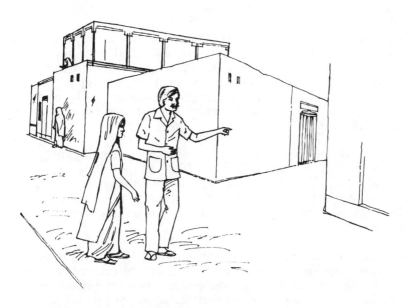

A community cannot be found simply by looking at the lines on a map. It is necessary to walk along the streets and talk to residents to discover where they consider the boundaries of their own community to be. The community survey (see pages 40–53) is an educational tool that will help you and the members of the community learn more about who belongs to the community and what are its special needs, resources, and culture.

Mr Jola's problem arose in a rural area. Health workers in towns and cities will find the same type of problem even more often. Towns are made up of many communities. A particular community may live in a certain neighbourhood, which may be divided from the next neighbourhood by streets or streams, but often is not.

Ask the residents to tell you who are the members of the different communities or neighbourhoods, and where they believe the boundary lines are located. Then each neighbourhood can be mobilized to identify and solve its own problems. There will be more cooperation and participation if the people feel that they belong together.

When is community health education needed?

Some health-related problems can be solved by individuals alone. To solve others, the cooperation of many people is needed. Here are some examples showing when the whole community needs to work together to solve a problem.

The provision of a clean water supply system requires time, labour, and materials. It is unlikely that each individual or family in a community can afford their own hygienic well. Similarly, if a village relies on one or two springs for its water supply, no one can have a private source. In that case, everyone in the community must cooperate in the building and maintenance of a protected spring.

In some villages people keep dogs for hunting, herding, or protection. These dogs often move freely in the village and may spread rabies. To increase the protection of the community, all dog-owners in the community must cooperate in immunizing their dogs against rabies. Everyone, not just dog-owners, would be concerned.

In times of emergency—for example, during floods—many families may lose supplies of food and clothing and be exposed to new health risks. All members of the community must come together and share what they have, so that the whole community will survive.

In short, community health education is needed when a problem affects many or all people in the community and when the cooperation of everyone is required to solve the problem.

How can you develop health education at community level? There are three points to keep in mind:

- You should get the support of influential people in the community, those who are called 'opinion leaders' or 'key people'.

- You should be sure that all the people of the community are informed about the problem and are kept up-to-date on plans and progress. All available channels of communication should be used for this purpose.

- You should get the maximum number of people involved so that the community will really strengthen its capacity to do things for its health. This can be done through community health committees, advisory or planning boards, etc.

We will now examine how we can go about achieving these objectives.

Getting opinion leaders involved

What is an opinion leader?

In every town or village there are people who are respected by others. They may be respected because of their ability to lead, because they are good at their profession (for example have a successful farm or business), because of their long experience, or because they are able to work well with certain groups such as women or young people. Some are very well known: religious and political leaders, for example. Some are quiet, but are respected because of their special wisdom or ability.

When people respect someone, they usually go to that person for advice. When respected people talk, other people listen. Respected people are called 'opinion leaders' because other people in the community value their opinions and ideas. Opinion leaders usually have a following. Not every opinion leader is respected by everyone in the village. Each section or group has its own opinion leaders.

Finding opinion leaders

Some opinion leaders have titles, which make them easy to identify. Examples of such titles are chief, counsellor, mayor, pastor, imam and reverend, and there are many others. The title alone does not make an opinion leader. Find out if a person with a title is popular within the political, religious, economic, or social group or organization. If, after talking to members of the group, you find out that the person is popular, then he or she is probably an opinion leader.

Since not all opinion leaders have titles, you should also look for them by asking people who they go to for advice on matters of concern (farming, child care, health, and other needs). If you find that many people name one individual, then you can be certain that this person is an opinion leader.

Working with opinion leaders

Visit the opinion leaders in your town. Find out their views on the welfare of the community. See what ideas they have about improving the community's health. Ask them for their advice. Share your own ideas with them and involve them in any local project. If they accept your ideas about community health, they may pass them on in advice to others. Opinion leaders have an important role in encouraging other people to adopt healthier behaviour and supporting them in their efforts to do so.

One thing to remember is that, since opinion leaders are usually elders or other important people, you should approach them in a respectful way. Let them know that you value their leadership in the community. If the leaders see that you respect them, they will listen to your ideas more closely.

The opinion leaders you will want to approach will depend on the type of programme. If your programme is about child health, visit the respected old grandmothers who influence child-raising practices. If you plan to develop a youth programme, look for youth leaders and young adults whom young people respect and listen to.

> Who are the important political, social, and religious opinion leaders in your village? Who are important opinion leaders among the farmers and the different craftsmen? Who are the important opinion leaders among the women?

The role of local organizations

Local organizations bring together people who have similar needs and interests. They can share ideas, give support to each other, and undertake projects together. Be sure to look for organizations that involve women, young people, and all other important sections of the community.

Local organizations vary in size depending on the number of people who have similar interests and want to be members. This could mean 10, 50, or more people. If there is a large number of members, they can divide into committees. Around 20 or 30 is a good number for carrying out projects, while still allowing participation.

Types of local organization

Branches of national organizations

There are many national and international organizations that encourage people to form local branches. Some examples are the Red Cross or Red Crescent Society, Boy and Girl Scouts or Guides, and the 4-H youth agricultural movement. The work of many of those groups is directly related to health and community development.

Local associations and clubs

These can be formed according to the particular needs and interests of people in your community. There may be a mothers' club at the preschool clinic. A fathers' club may also be organized to educate and involve fathers in the care and needs of their children. Children themselves can form health clubs.

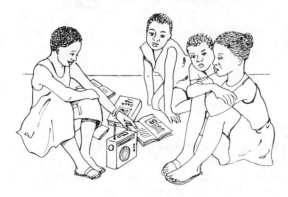

Children at their health club.

We saw in Chapter 5, pages 131–134, how patients with a long-term illness, namely diabetes, found it useful to form a club. At a school there could be many different clubs based on the different interests of pupils, such as science and drama. Parents with handicapped children could get together in an association to see how best to cope with problems of the children's education. A group of citizens could form an association to deal with problems related to a major local disease or to protect the environment.

Starting a local organization

Finding needs

Look around your clinic, schools, and community. Are there people with special needs and interests? Would they be able to solve their problems better if they worked together in an association?

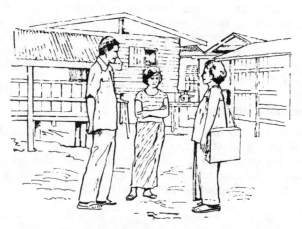

If there is no organization in the community to cope with a specific need you have identified, you may want to start one. Talk to people, especially community leaders, to see if it is a good idea. Often, there is already an organization that can extend its activity to meet the need.

Encouraging interest

Talk to people. Find out what they have been doing to solve their problems. Do they need the support and encouragement of others? Explain the value and purpose of organizing an association or a club. Find out if people would be willing to meet with others to discuss such a project.

Holding an exploratory meeting

Hold a meeting where people can explore the idea. At the meeting explain the idea again. Encourage people to ask questions. Make sure they understand clearly.

Do not push the idea too hard. People may become suspicious or uncooperative if it looks as though you are trying to force them. There will always be some people who have doubts. They will ask questions like, 'Will I have to pay for anything?' 'Who will be in charge?' Answer all questions politely and completely.

Clarifying responsibilities

During the exploratory meeting and afterwards, always make it clear to the group that the association or the club they form belongs to them and that they will make all the decisions about activities. The purpose is that people should be better organized to help themselves.

Explain that your role will be to serve as advisor or guide. You are not the leader. You do not give directions. You are there to help members do whatever they want to do.

Deciding to begin

At some point during the first exploratory meeting, or at follow-up meetings, a decision will be reached on whether to establish a formal group or not. This is a decision that those who are interested must make for themselves.

Do not be surprised if most of the people react positively about the project, but a few do not. Not all hypertensive patients will want to share their problems with others. Not every father would want to belong to a fathers' club.

Encourage those who are interested to go ahead. Let the others know that they are welcome to join whenever they have the time and inclination.

Setting up a structure for the organization

For an association or a club to work well over months and years, it needs a structure. That means that there should be leaders, a clearly stated purpose, and a few rules or procedures.

These are all issues and decisions that the members of the group should work out for themselves. You should encourage them to set things up in the way that feels most familiar and comfortable to them. Do not tell them that they must have a chairperson, a treasurer, and a secretary. Explain that it is a usual procedure to have some form of leadership as this is helpful for getting things done. In the case of a branch of a national association, it may even be obligatory to have a specific leadership structure. See with the people what fits best into the local culture.

You can ask general questions to help the members think: 'What do you want to do about leadership?' 'Is everyone clear about the purpose of the club?' Refer to the section on meetings at the end of Chapter 5 for more information on conducting such a session. Encourage understanding, participation and consensus.

Make it clear to people that any formal group needs to have activities and projects or its members will lose interest. If there are regular meeting-times, members can work together on activities that will help solve problems faced by everyone.

The community health committee

One way to achieve community involvement is to encourage the establishment of health committees. Their members will help you to know what the people feel are their priority needs, and in turn you can guide them towards appropriate action. Let us see in more detail what is the purpose of a health committee and how it can be established.

Purpose of a health committee

It is difficult to imagine 50 or 100 people meeting together to plan the details of a community health programme. Not everyone would get a chance to speak. Much time would be spent trying to make sure that everyone understood and participated. Some people would not want to waste time and would possibly try to force the group to make quick decisions. This might make others angry and then arguments would start.

In order to avoid these problems, smaller groups called committees are often chosen. The committee is given a specific task or job. It carries out that task and then reports back to the larger group with some suggestions for action. The committee's investigations and plans make it easier and quicker for the larger group to make decisions.

Although every individual, family, and group in the community is responsible for health, as we have said before, it is often useful to have an organized group—a committee—whose special purpose is to reflect the needs of the people and to help the community look after its health. Each community would need to decide on the exact duties of its own health committee, but here are some general tasks on which a health committee would work:

● Collecting information about the health of the community.

● Identifying community health problems and the reasons for them.

● Proposing solutions and plans for solving the problems.

● Discussing these solutions and plans with the health workers who will help them (*a*) decide on priorities, (*b*) develop realistic goals, and (*c*) locate resources.

● Mobilizing the community to achieve the goals set and solve its own problems.

● Keeping the community up-to-date on progress and on problems encountered.

Establishing a health committee

First, you must find out if the community sees a need for a group to look especially into health and related problems. The idea needs to be thoroughly discussed with community members and leaders. They must decide for themselves whether or not they want a health committee. If they do, the committee can either be formed within an existing group or be a completely new body.

There may already be groups in the community that are concerned with, and responsible for, the health and development of the community. It is easier to work with existing groups if the people in the community accept these groups and are satisfied with the work that they have been doing. If there are too many committees and groups, especially if they are doing similar things, time and resources are wasted and people will lose interest.

Perhaps there is already a large village or community council that is involved in many activities. Such a council may not have time to look at health matters, in which case several of its members could be nominated to form a health committee that would report back to the larger council for final decisions.

If there is no existing group that could serve as a base, then a new committee could be formed. There are several steps to follow in forming a new committee.

First, who shall be the members? If the committee is to be helpful to the community, it must contain people who are respected and who are willing to work hard for the improvement of their community. Another thing to consider is whether the health committee will be able to look after the interests of all sections and groups in the community. A community is often made up of different professional, political, religious, and other groups. If one group or section of the community is left out of the health committee, people belonging to that group may not cooperate on a community health programme suggested by the committee.

Secondly, how do you select committee members? Remember that each community has its own culture and ways of doing things. There are many possible ways of selecting health committee members. Three are listed here:

- Hold a community meeting where members could be nominated, appointed, or elected, or could volunteer, whichever way is acceptable.

- Community leaders could appoint the people they feel are best for the job.

- The various interest groups in the community could be asked to select people to represent them on the committee.

Think of other ways to establish a health committee, and follow the one that is most likely to be acceptable to people in your community. If members are not selected in an acceptable way, people will not respect the work of the committee. It would probably be helpful for any health committee to include people who practise either traditional or modern medicine.

The next question to consider is: how many members should the committee have? A health committee should be large enough to represent the main interests in the community, but small enough for all the members to participate, discuss, and work together easily. The ideal number of members might be around ten.

Finally, to whom does a health committee report? The committee should report regularly to the community leaders on its activities and progress. It should also be constantly in touch with health workers to inform them of problems and plans and to obtain guidance and support from them. The committee should be open to ideas and suggestions and to receiving help from any members of the community at any time.

Promoting participation

From your experience you probably know that it is often difficult to obtain the participation of every member, even in small groups. Participation by the whole community is still more difficult. Here are some reasons people may give for not participating in a community project.

- 'No one told me about the project.'

- 'I was angry: they only told me a few days in advance.'

- 'They never thanked me for the work I did the last time.'

- 'I did not agree with the plan.'

- 'The date was the same as the big market in the district town, so we couldn't come.'

- 'No one told me exactly what I was supposed to do.'

- 'They never asked me what I thought, so why should I help?'

Have you heard other reasons being given for not participating?

To encourage participation, you should try to:

- Keep people informed about activities that are being planned.

- Encourage suggestions to be made, directly or through a representative, to the planning committee.

- Set out specific tasks and jobs for everyone. You will need to explain the tasks and maybe provide some training. People should also understand how important their own job is to the success of the whole project.

- Find out on what date most people will be able to participate.

- Give praise and show appreciation to all who help. For example you could take a photograph of everyone who helped with a project and display it where it can be seen by members of the community.

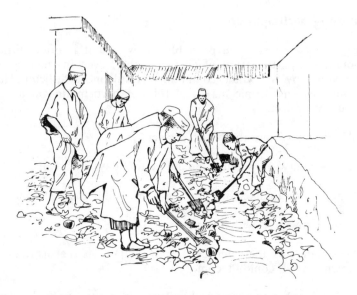

For a community-wide clean-up campaign to be successful, individuals, groups, and whole neighbourhoods must participate. Efforts should be made to see that the clean-up activities continue throughout the year.

Advisory and planning boards

A community health facility such as a health centre or clinic, should be designed to meet the needs of the people in the community. The services it offers should continue to be seen as useful to the community.

Community participation

There must be some means by which people in the community can give not only their views and suggestions, but also participate in making decisions about the design and running of the services.

One way to make sure community views are heard and considered is to organize an advisory and planning board made up of citizens who make use of the services.

An existing group or committee could serve this purpose. If a new group needs to be formed, follow the general suggestions given for forming a health committee. The members of the board must be willing to work. They should gather good background information about problems before they make suggestions.

Views of health workers

Health workers often feel uncomfortable when community members offer suggestions and criticisms about the health service. They feel that the community does not appreciate their hard work. This is not usually the case. People in the community simply want what they think is the best for themselves and their children.

An advisory board will not work unless the health staff welcomes the idea as much as the community does. Meetings, discussions, and even individual counselling with health staff on the subject of community participation may be necessary. Health service staff themselves may need education on the value and meaning of participation as we have described it in this book (see particularly, Chapter 2, pages 32–36).

Training board members

The members of the community who serve on an advisory or planning board need training so that they can do their jobs well and communicate easily with the staff.

Communication skills

The board members will appreciate it if health workers use simple language that they can easily understand and if they explain to them the meaning of some of the technical terms or special words that health workers use. They will then be better able to understand what is being discussed at meetings. Board members also need to feel that they are welcome to ask questions.

Collecting information

If board members know how to collect accurate information about the health problems of their community and the possible causes of these problems, they will be able to give health staff better suggestions about improving services.

Running a board meeting

Ways of running meetings are different in different cultures. The health staff may also have its own way of running meetings. When the health staff and board members get together for a meeting, they must agree on how they will run the meeting; how permission will be given to speak; how decisions will be made; what kind of leadership there will be; and other issues.

Whatever training sessions you may organize, you must remember that board members and health staff must have good relations if they are to work together. Informal gatherings can be planned so that members and staff get to know each other socially. Small-group and one-to-one discussion can also help.

Taking action

Board members should take time to explain and discuss their views with health workers until everyone sees a clear line of action. Then they must be willing to work with the health workers to be sure that changes and improvements are made as desired.

Contact with the community

Just like a health committee, an advisory board serves the community leaders and members. The board should meet with community groups and leaders to share what they learn about the health service. In a way, such a board is a link between the community and the health service.

Intersectoral coordination groups

So far we have only talked about health staff and groups. There are many other people who work for community improvement and health: agricultural agents, social welfare workers, community development officers, schoolteachers, adult education teachers, and others. Those people should be involved as much as possible in all health programmes, and health workers should in turn be involved in the programmes of the other community workers and their agencies. Another important group to involve are people working for the mass media (radio broadcasters, newspaper repo-rters, etc.), should such people be available in your community.

Before such involvement can be successful, there must be good communication between all the different agencies. The formation of a community services council is one way of promoting communication and cooperation. This council could meet regularly, maybe once a month or more frequently, should the need arise. Each agency would send some representatives. General community needs could be discussed and the roles and responsibilities of each agency could be planned.

Skills in holding meetings and encouraging mature group behaviour will be most important for the success of such a council. Each agency will feel that its job in the community is very important. People in one agency may not trust people in others. There may have been disagreements in the past. Hard work may be needed to build good relationships. The time and effort will be worthwhile, because the members of the community will benefit through better services.

Before setting up a new structure—be it a health committee, an advisory board, a local association, or a council to facilitate intersectoral coordination—investigate carefully the structures that already exist in the community and see if they could serve for the purpose you envisage. It is often tempting to create a new group but it may be wiser to extend an organization that has proved its worth.

Organizing a health campaign

Purpose

Campaigns can be planned to promote knowledge, skills, attitudes, and values relating to a particular health issue. They may also be used to accomplish a particular community improvement project.

Public awareness is the first key to a successful health campaign. Therefore a carefully planned public information programme should begin as soon as the community decides on the issue or problem it wants to tackle. People need to know what is going to happen, when it will happen, and why the project is important to them. In the course of the campaign, this information is provided through a series of messages, for which every available channel of communication is used, including personal outreach, town criers, posters, public address systems, announcements at public or group meeting places, and, if possible, radio and newspaper coverage.

A health campaign is organized around one issue or problem. In other words, it has a theme. Examples of themes are 'Clean up the community', 'Immunize your child', 'Good food for healthy bodies', 'Clean water for good health'. These themes will often become the name of the campaign, so should be short, 'catchy', and easy to remember.

The campaign should be concerned with a real problem that has been identified by the community members themselves or is generally recognized. If there is a health committee in the community, it should be active in identifying subjects for campaigns and planning appropriate action.

The duration of the actual campaign activities in the community is often only a week or a month. For this reason, campaigns are often known as 'Health weeks'.

Advanced planning

While the campaign itself may last only one week, it must be preceded by much planning. The committee may work for several months or a year in order to plan a successful campaign and the necessary follow-up. Members of the community must be contacted well in advance, if they are expected to participate in projects and donate money and materials. Resources must be located, and educational activities organized.

The use of a variety of health education methods will help reinforce the impact. There may be plays, health talks, displays, demonstrations, community meetings, and group discussions. Programmes may be organized in the schools and with other community groups.

Opportunities are provided for the community to participate in projects such as digging latrine pits or building incinerators.

Follow-up

An activity that lasts for a week creates much excitement and interest. But health problems are not solved if people are active for only one week out of the year. They must practise healthy behaviour throughout the year. They must help maintain community wells and latrines in good order every day, not just on one day.

If a health committee exists, its members must watch to see if people continue to practise the health skills taught during the campaign. Home visits, community meetings, posters, group discussions, and school projects throughout the year help people to remember the knowledge and practise the skills they have learnt, and also to maintain the health facilities they have created.

The need for follow-up is one reason why campaigns should be organized by the community itself (through its committees or councils), and not by health workers alone. Follow-up activities are carried out most effectively by the people who live in the community.

For example, a one-week campaign on immunization would be useless without adequate follow-up. Several immunizations require second doses three months after the first. Also, new babies require

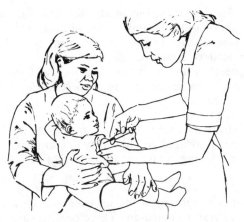

This child is being immunized as part of a campaign. For the campaign to be successful, planned follow-up is needed.

immunization at different times throughout the year. Planned follow-up activities are therefore essential to make sure that the campaign succeeds in its health objectives.

Special community events

Every community has festivals, celebrations, and ceremonies. These may mark special seasons of the year such as harvest time, the planting season, or the new year. Some festivals are religious or political, others are held in remembrance of national events and heroes. There are usually many such events throughout the year.

Some festivals are a time for enjoyment and relaxation. Others call for serious thinking and quiet devotion. Whatever the purpose of the festival may be, the whole community usually participates.

Educational value

Most community events have some connection with the health and welfare of the community. A harvest or thanksgiving festival is a time for enjoying and appreciating the bounty of the earth. It can also be a time to think about such things as:

- Nutrition.
- Food storage.
- What use to make of profits.
- How to plan for a better crop next season.

The high level of interest and excitement found during festivals and celebrations can be focused on these issues, which are all related to health. Health education in the form of drama, song, dance, displays, school projects and group discussion can be planned for the time of the festival. If the event is political or religious, opinion leaders could be asked to refer to health concerns in the speeches and sermons. During the festival period, special activities could be organized by schoolchildren for their schools and their parents.

Talks and demonstrations could be given at the clinic. Let people know that the topic is related to the festival taking place. Use traditional dancing, singing, plays, story-telling, and other forms of art.

Planning educational programmes for an event or festival is much like planning for a health campaign. Therefore be sure that the community groups and committees participate in the selection and planning of the educational activities. Again, as in campaigns, community participation is necessary to guarantee follow-up which will ensure that people's new ideas and skills are not lost.

> What are some of the festivals and events in your community? How is each festival related to health or community development? What kind of educational activities could be useful in each festival? Who are some of the local opinion leaders, artists, and community workers that could assist in educational programmes?

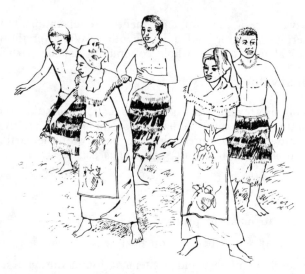

A community festival.

Mobilizing community resources for a project

Mobilizing community resources means that every member of the community is encouraged to give whatever resources he or she can offer towards solving a community problem. A health committee, club, or association cannot build a new market, a road, or a well alone. Help is needed from the whole community.

Planning the project

The planning skills described in Chapter 3 are most useful here. One of the main things to remember is that the community should:

- Identify its own needs.

- Plan its own solutions.

- Get the maximum number of people to participate voluntarily in the project.

A main purpose is to strengthen the ability of people to solve their problems using their own resources. Besides being the least costly way of solving a problem, using local resources also gives

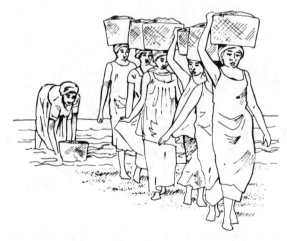

People in this village have decided to build a new classroom for their primary school through self-help. Here the village women are participating by collecting sand, a local resource to be used in making cement for the building.

people a feeling of pride and self-worth. Identifying resources (pages 64–71) is most important for the effective mobilization of the community.

You should not make plans for the group. Encourage its members to make decisions for themselves. Decision-making is one of the skills the group is learning. Of course you may give guidance and suggestions. In particular, make sure the group is realistic about the amount of time and other resources they will need for the project.

Developing self-reliance

As the group begins the project, you should be around to watch and give suggestions. You may have to demonstrate some new skills. Then step back and let the people learn by doing the work for themselves. As the work is being done, meet the people and discuss their progress. Find out what they are learning. Praise them when they are doing well.

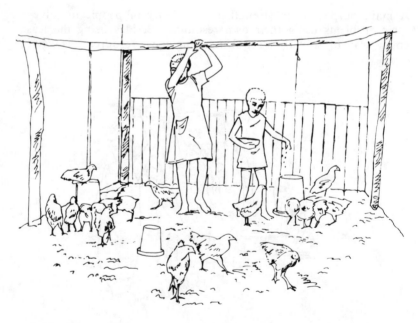

A school-run poultry farm is a project through which children can learn about nutrition, develop a sense of responsibility and gain self-help skills, and therefore self-reliance. These skills and the feeling of self-reliance will spread to the families of the children.

Point out any problems you might see. Ask the group to think of solutions to the problems.

At the end, discuss with the person or group the results they have achieved. Find out if they are happy with the way the project turned out. What new skills and ideas did they learn? What might they do better next time? Praise them for what they have achieved. This will encourage them to continue.

If a project does not succeed, people often become sad or angry. This is natural. If this happens, you must help people see that learning can come out of mistakes too. Help them see the reasons for the failure. Do not let people start blaming each other. Encourage them to discuss how they will work better next time.

> Think about the values in the community where you work. Do people value cooperation and helping friends in need? Do they value the idea of each person giving service to the community? Is it important to people that their community looks progressive to the neighbouring communities?

If these values are present in a community, people are likely to be motivated into action that will improve their community and develop self-reliance.

Developing a partnership with people

People do not always understand why they should try to improve their health by their own efforts. They feel sometimes that health care is the responsibility of the government. Of course, the government has a responsibility in this area. And it is clear that the promotion of people's self-reliance should in no way be an excuse for health workers to avoid rendering the services that the community is entitled to receive.

Here is an example of a community-based project where it took a long time to establish a real partnership.

> Right from the beginning, the health project workers tried to involve the people in planning and programming. They were careful to ask 'What can we do together about the problem?', and they started defining the issues with the

people. The people liked this very much, because they had an input to make. Previously, in another development project in the area, health workers had been conducting surveys without consulting them. The people did not even know what happened to the surveys afterwards. There was no feedback whatsoever. So, this time, they really appreciated being involved and informed.

However, when the point of planning was reached and the health workers asked 'What can you do about your problem?', the people were shocked.

They said 'Why us, why not you? It is your duty.' They had been quite comfortable letting health workers take action in the past. Now they were asked to do something about their problems themselves. The people did not quite understand why it should be that way.

The leader of the project said that one important lesson they learned was that they needed to help people regain confidence in themselves and to reassure them that they could do it. She explained that in the past, health workers had taken away from the people their decision-making power and discouraged them from thinking for themselves. This led to people lacking confidence in their capacity to become active partners.

Partnership, self-reliance and community participation are all easy to discuss in a forum. They are much more difficult to put into practice. As the saying goes, 'it is easier said than done'. Involving the community requires a tremendous investment of human resources, time and effort. No health worker can make an effective investment without commitment and motivation.

What sustained the project workers through the difficult moments at the beginning was a belief in people. The project workers gave the community much more than expertise, and technical knowledge – they were totally committed to making the project work. When the people realized this a positive relationship started to grow.

Now the project is developing very well and the people are very much involved.

Think about your own experience. Have you sometimes found people reluctant to make an effort or to take on certain responsibilities to improve their health? What were the reasons? Did you have the skills necessary to take action? Had you been teaching them these skills?

In what circumstances did you find people most willing to cooperate? What were the factors that created this partnership between you and them?

The role of the community health worker

One of the most important ways of providing health education to a community is through the selection and training of community health workers.

Functions of a community health worker

The community health worker comes from the community and is trained to work in it, in close relationship with the health care system. The community health worker is expected to perform a wide range of functions, which generally include: home visits, environmental sanitation, provision of an adequate and safe water supply, first aid and treatment of simple and common ailments, health education, nutritional surveillance, maternal and child health and family planning activities, communicable diseases control, community development activities, referrals, record-keeping, and collection of data on vital events.

These functions have been shaped to a large extent by the Declaration of Alma-Ata, which outlined the eight essential components of primary health care as being: education concerning prevailing health problems and the methods of preventing and controlling them; promotion of food supply and proper nutrition: an adequate supply of safe water and basic sanitation; maternal and child health care, including family planning; immunization against the major infectious diseases; prevention and control of locally endemic diseases; appropriate treatment of common diseases and injuries; and provision of essential drugs.

Community health workers are in a unique position because they have a role both in the community and within the health care system. They make a bridge between one and the other. In the community they help to identify problems, and people at risk or in need. They involve the community in planning how to deal with its own problems, and they help the community to be in touch with the health services. The community health worker also provides the health services with the information needed for surveillance, planning, and management.

Training and supervision

The training and supervision of community health workers are among the primary health care tasks in which health education has a major part to play. Through health education, we must make sure that the community is involved in selecting its health workers. Through discussion with the trainees, we should agree on a time and place that is convenient for the training. Local communication and education methods should be used in the training to aid understanding. Trainers should learn how the local culture views health, and specific diseases, so that local beliefs and customs can be effectively discussed during training.

The community health worker acts as a 'bridge' between the community and the health services, and plays a key role in helping the community express its needs and develop self-reliance.

The concept of the community health worker is an important advance in finding ways to make health care accessible to all.

Many, if not most, community health workers are volunteers. They may be paid little or nothing for their work. They need regular support from supervisory staff, such as a community nurse or public health inspector, to help them keep up their morale. The supervisors should help the community health workers remember their tasks. They should also help inform the community about the community health workers' jobs and encourage the community to support their work. We should be careful not to expect too much from community health workers who are volunteers. We should give them constant encouragement and praise when it is due, because without these workers at the grassroots level there would be no primary health care.

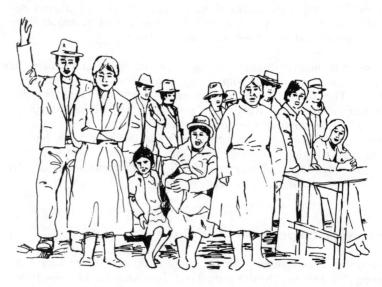

A villager volunteers to be a health worker.

Chapter 7

Communicating the health message: methods and media

As we have seen, health education helps people to make wise choices about their health and the quality of life of their community. To do this, accurate information must be presented in an understandable form. Often many different presentations of the same facts and ideas are needed.

In this chapter methods, media, and techniques that can be used to communicate health messages are discussed. Suggestions are given for developing and using each approach. The chapter cannot cover all methods. You can probably think of other ways of informing and educating the people around you. In fact, the better you know the local people, the more likely you are to develop the best ways of communicating with them. There are two different ways to put across health messages. The first is the direct person-to-person method where you, the health worker, are the principal communicator. The second is the indirect method, in which your role is to convey to your local audience health messages that originate elsewhere, for example radio and television programmes. This classification into two groups is very general, and there is often overlap. Posters, for example, may be considered as an indirect method when they are simply put on a noticeboard in a health centre. They can also complement direct methods when they are used as part of a health talk. Indirect methods can originate within or outside the local community. Locally produced materials will be particularly relevant but you can make outside materials more effective for your community by the way you use and interpret them.

The important thing to remember is that effective health communication is seldom achieved through the use of one method alone, or even two or three methods. Your success will depend on your ability to combine a variety of methods, both person-to-person and indirect, to accomplish your educational purpose. You are working at the critical point where the media meet the people.

Communicating the health message

The nature and role of communication

We have seen in Chapter 2 that health education is people working with people to solve problems and improve the quality of life. Communication helps to equip people with the facts, ideas and attitudes they need to make informed decisions about their health.

Communication occurs when a message is transmitted and received. The message in health education is something that it is considered important for the people in the community to know or do. The source may be a local health worker or a national government, or members of the community may themselves recognize a need for change. The message may be transmitted person-to-person in private conversation, or in a group meeting or health talk, or indirectly by a radio broadcast or newspaper.

The important thing is what happens when the message reaches the people it is aimed at. If they hear and understand it, and are inclined to believe it, good communication has taken place.

Communication alone rarely changes behaviour. As we have seen, behaviour is too complex for that. But facts or ideas that are heard, understood and believed are necessary to pave the way for desired changes in behaviour and informed community participation.

Some prerequisites to efficient communication

Chapter 3, pages 74–80, was devoted to the selection of appropriate methods as part of the process of planning in health education. Once a number of basic questions concerning the people, the resources, the local circumstances and culture have been examined, further questions still remain to be answered. They concern how to put educational methods into practice, and the need to pre-test methods and materials.

Putting educational methods into practice

There are three things to consider when putting educational methods into use:

- When to find people.

- Where to find people.

- How to involve people.

Choose the right time

For example when working with farmers, find out when they work and when they rest. Women normally have certain times when they work at home or away from home, and when they go to the market. A meeting or a discussion with women must be planned for when they have free time. If a display is to be set up in the market, it must be done when people are gathered there. For education with children, you must know when they are at school, when they are helping their parents and when they are free. Get together with the people concerned and plan a time for the educational programme that is best for everyone.

Choose a convenient place

Find out where people normally gather—markets, schools, work-places, churches, mosques or temples. There are also places where people gather socially. There may be a small community building that is used for important meetings. People may also gather in front of the chief's house or the houses of other important leaders. You and the group can decide which is the easiest place for everyone to reach.

Involve people

There are many ways to do this. Some methods like plays and discussions require more participation than others. But even when you give a talk or show a film, you can always find ways to get the people involved by asking questions or getting them to do things themselves. Promoting participation is very important because people learn better when they are not passive. Ways to get them involved will be discussed with each method.

Pre-testing

Before we put an educational method into practice, or use educational materials, we should make sure that they are well suited to the situation and to the group, otherwise they will not have the impact desired. So pre-testing is needed whenever possible. Pre-testing means trying out an educational method with a small group of people. If the method works in the way that you hoped, then you can use it with other people and groups in the community.

Methods and materials that need pre-testing are those that are prepared in advance, such as stories, fables, songs, posters, flip-charts, flannelgraphs, plays, puppet shows, films, slides and photographs. Not all methods can be pre-tested because not all can be prepared in advance. For example, with role-play, meetings, and discussion groups, there may be a general idea of the topic in advance, but these methods only work if the

199

participants make up the action and decisions as they go along. In other words, people must be free to act creatively.

It is necessary to pre-test methods and materials. First, people may not understand the purpose of the method. Second, they may not understand the message you are trying to share. Third, they may not like what they see or hear. If, for example, a poster does not look attractive, people may ignore it. If you can find out the problems people have in understanding your methods, you can change and improve them. Your educational methods will be more effective if you can make improvements before you begin your programme. Here are the steps you can follow for pre-testing.

Prepare your materials well

Look at them yourself to see if they are clear and simple. Correct any mistakes.

Gather the group for the pre-test

Choose people who are similar to the people who will use the finished materials. If you will be showing posters to mothers at a pre-school clinic, gather four or five of these mothers together to help you pre-test. If you are preparing a story for farmers, bring a few farmers together to listen to you.

Present the materials

Allow the small group to see or hear what you have prepared.

Ask questions

Find out whether the group has understood and accepted what you presented. If you were testing a poster, here are examples of the types of questions you might ask.

- What do you think is the message or the idea in this poster?

- Who do you think this poster is planned for (adults, children, men, women, farmers, workers, etc.)?

- What would your friends think if they saw this poster?

- Do you think the poster could look nicer? Do you think the poster is planned for people living in this village/town/area?

- Do you think other colours should be used?

- Are the pictures, drawings and words big enough, too big or too small?

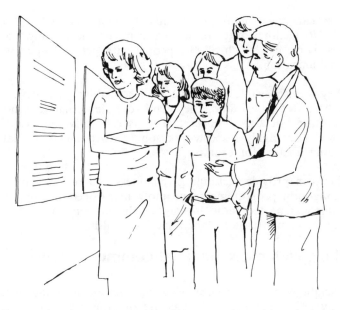

Asking questions is an important part of the pre-testing and use of educational methods. Through asking questions, you will learn whether a method is acceptable and makes sense to people.

- In what ways do you think the poster could be improved?

- Are the ideas and suggestions on the poster practical and useful?

Make changes

Be prepared to change your materials according to the suggestions you have received.

Using mass media

When we hear the term mass media we tend to think of something huge and impersonal—a newspaper printed on giant presses in the national capital, a radio broadcast for millions of listeners or, a television programme produced at enormous cost. But 'mass' media need not be 'big' media. In many places there are newspapers serving small towns and rural areas. Many small cities have local radio stations. It is true, of course, that not everyone can read, and that many people do not own a radio. But the numbers reached by these media are growing each year. These media, used as part of a health communication plan, have great advantages.

- They can reach many people quickly. Our goal is 'Health for all'. No health worker or health team, no matter how hard they work, can reach all the people with person-to-person communication.

- They are believable. If people read something in a newspaper or hear it on the radio, they tend to believe that it is not only true but also important. This is especially the case if the 'voice' is a highly respected person—a government official or a leading doctor, for example.

- They can provide continuing reminders and reinforcement. In a long-term programme to promote breast-feeding, for example, repeated radio messages help mothers to remember why it is important for their babies' health.

Working with mass media at community level

As a health worker in a rural village or urban neighbourhood, you may feel that the mass media are of little use to you. This is not necessarily true. These media can add such strength to an education programme that you should explore every possibility of working with them.

Find out about the media in your area

If people in your community read a newspaper, which paper do they read? Remember, even if only a few people read newspapers, they are likely to be opinion leaders. Where is this newspaper printed? If it is printed in a nearby town, who writes the news about your district? Is there someone who writes about health? Would these people be interested in a story about a local health event?

Ask the same kind of questions about radio. What programmes do the men or women listen to? At what times of day do the people listen most? Do all the programmes come from the capital city? Are there regular programmes about health? If there is a radio station in or near your district, would it be willing to broadcast your immunization schedule, for example?

Be aware of media health coverage

Even if you find that you are not able to use radio or news-papers for your own messages, you can still use mass media in your education programme. To do so effectively you must first be aware of the health-related stories covered by the media.

In the case of newspapers, be especially alert for stories in which your country's President or Minister of Health makes a statement concerning health. This happens more often than you might think. If, for example, the President proclaims a national campaign against polio, cut out the article, put it up in a prominent place, and be prepared to answer questions about it. Use the article as the basis for a community or health committee meeting on the topic.

Radio stations often print or announce their schedule or programmes in advance. If you find out that a programme on health is planned for a certain day and time, invite a group of people to listen together and discuss the topic afterwards. Again, prepare yourself to answer questions. These 'radio meetings' are an ideal way to combine the benefits of person-to-person and media communication.

Methods and media

Health talks

Purpose

The most natural way of communicating with people is to talk with them. In health education, we have many opportunities to talk with people. We may do this with one person or with a family, with a small group or with many people together. Health talks have been, and remain, the most common way to share health knowledge and facts. Too often, however, this method is used by itself. Talk alone is too much like giving advice. As mentioned in Chapters 1 and 4, advice is not the same as health education.

To make a talk more educational, it must be combined with other methods, especially visual aids, such as posters, slides, and flannelgraphs. A talk should be tied into the local setting by the use of proverbs, for example. Interaction and interest should be aroused by using discussion, songs and possibly role-plays and demonstrations.

Group size

Talks are usually given to small gatherings, although they are sometimes given to much larger groups. For example, a talk broadcast over the radio may reach everyone in the country.

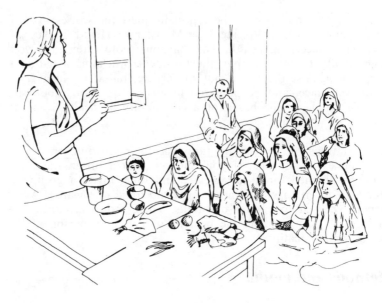

When a health talk is well prepared and presented in a lively way, it is an effective method of sharing health knowledge and facts.

Participation

One problem is that the larger the group, the less participation and discussion are possible. Discussion is necessary so that people can ask questions, share ideas, and be clear about the real message of the talk. This is easy in small groups of 5 to 10 people. In larger groups there is less chance for each person to ask his or her own questions. After hearing a talk to a larger group, some people may go away confused. One way to solve this problem, is for you to stay after the talk so that people can come to you individually to ask their questions.

With talks on the radio, it is not possible to ask questions of the speaker. This problem can be solved by holding a radio meeting (see pages 242–243). Participation and discussion help you learn too. You learn how well you are able to communicate. If many people understand your points, then you are a good speaker. If not, you should try to find out why, and then try to do better.

Do not accept silence as agreement or understanding. Ask the group questions to be sure that they understand your points.

Preparing a talk

The following points must be considered carefully.

Know the group

Find out their needs and interests.

Select an appropriate topic

This should be a single, simple topic. Nutrition is too big as a topic. It would take weeks to talk about all the aspects of nutrition. Nutrition can be broken down into many simple topics, such as breast-feeding, weaning diet, body-building foods, food needs of older people, cooking methods that preserve food value, etc.

Have correct and up-to-date information

Check in your books and consult resource people (your supervisor perhaps) to check that all your facts are accurate.

List the points you will make

There should only be a few main points. People may forget if you tell them too many things.

Write down what you will say

If you do not like writing, you must think carefully about what to include in your talk. Think of examples, proverbs and stories to help emphasize your points.

Think of visual aids

Well chosen posters, photos, etc., will help people learn.

Practise your whole talk

This should include the telling of stories and the showing of posters and pictures.

How many minutes does your talk take?

The whole talk, including showing visual aids, should take about 15 to 20 minutes. You should allow another 15 minutes or more for questions and discussion. If the talk is too long people may become bored and restless.

Making arrangements

Good organization demands that you pay attention to many details.

Where will you give the talk?

Is the place free from noise? If it is the rainy season, is the place protected from the weather? Is there room for the whole group to gather comfortably? Are there enough seats for those who need them? Is the place small enough for people at the back of the group to hear and see? Can everyone get to the place easily?

At what time will you give the talk

Pick a time when the people in the group have no other duties. Do not pick a time that conflicts with another community event.

A talk may be given at a regular meeting of a social, religious or other organization in the community. Find out the schedule or agenda for those meetings. Do not take more time than the group offers you. They may have other important business to conduct.

Proverbs

Proverbs are short common-sense sayings that are handed down from generation to generation. They grow out of the experiences of people in each culture. They are like advice on how best to behave.

Some proverbs are straightforward—their meaning is obvious. Others are more complicated. The listener has to think carefully in order to understand them. Here are some proverbs from a country in Africa. See if you can understand their meaning.

(a) One does not go in search of a cure for ringworm while leaving leprosy unattended.

(b) A young man may have as many new clothes, but not as many worn-out clothes, as an old man.

(c) A hen drinks water, swallows pebbles, but still complains she has no teeth. Does a goat with many teeth eat iron?

Purpose

Proverbs can support or illustrate a point about health you want to get across.

Discovering local proverbs

You may already know many proverbs from the village or community where you work. If you do not, the best way to learn proverbs is to talk with the older people. They may even help you with your educational programmes, because they often enjoy telling proverbs.

Educational use

Proverbs can be combined with talks, demonstrations, stories, dramas, or put on posters and flipcharts. Think of other uses. People are very familiar with their proverbs. When you use a proverb correctly, people will be impressed that you understand their culture. Since the proverb is familiar, they may try to abide by the advice it gives in relation to health.

Here are the meanings of the three proverbs.

(*a*) Try to solve the most serious problem first.

(*b*) An old man has more experience than a young one.

(*c*) Some people have what they need but are still not content.

The first proverb could be useful during a talk to mothers that emphasizes the importance of bringing their children to the clinic when they are sick, instead of going about some other business.

The second proverb could encourage young people to respect and care for their elderly parents.

The last proverb could remind people to be realistic when they plan a project.

If you are with a group of health or community workers, ask each one to tell you a traditional proverb. Discuss each proverb. See how it can be used to help communicate ideas about health.

Fables

Fables are make-believe stories that have been told to children for generations. The characters in a fable are often animals.

Purpose

The actions of the characters in a fable are supposed to teach children proper ways of behaving. Fables also show adults what values are important to the community.

Group size

Fables can be used with individuals or small groups. They can also be used in radio programmes that reach a large number of people.

A sample fable

The tortoise is an animal that often appears in fables. Children always listen carefully to this fable to find out if the tortoise will solve the problem.

The tortoise and the goat were good friends. They often took long walks together. One day while they were walking, the goat said: 'I fancy something nice to eat. Let's find some food.' The tortoise agreed and they began searching. Soon they could smell some delicious food cooking. They followed the smell to the lion's house. They looked around and saw that the lion was far away from his house. The tortoise said, 'There is a small door in the back of the house. We can go in quietly, eat quickly, and then escape through that small door. The lion will never catch us.' They squeezed themselves through the small back door and began feasting on the lion's supper. The tortoise ate a little and was satisfied, but the goat continued to eat and eat. Soon they looked up and saw the lion returning. They rushed to the small back door. The tortoise slipped through the door easily, but the goat was so full of food that he could only get halfway through. He got stuck. The tortoise tried to pull him out but it did no good.

When the lion came into his house he was very hungry. He said, 'I need my supper but someone has eaten nearly all of it, and there is that fat someone trying to escape through my back door.' He pulled the fat goat into the house. Since the lion didn't have any other food he decided to make goat-meat stew for his supper. By this time the tortoise had run far away. He realized that he had only escaped because he hadn't eaten too much food, but also that the lion needed his food because he was hungry. He decided he would never take another person's food again.

From this fable children would learn not to steal and not to be greedy.

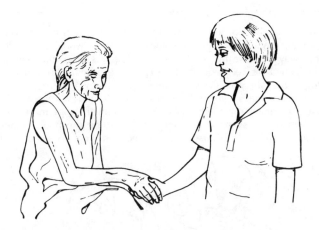

Many useful fables can be learned by talking with elderly people, who can also tell you much about the history, culture, and problems of the community.

Educational use

Fables are useful when you are talking to small groups of children. They are also useful for health education with parents. The parents will then be able to tell the fable to their own children. After telling a fable you should always discuss it with those who listened. Ask questions. Why did the goat eat the lion's food? Was this a good thing to do? Why did the lion eat the goat? Was the decision the tortoise made at the end a good one? By encouraging people to think about and discuss the story, you will help them learn. Ask people to tell their own fables too. See if they can make one up about health.

A fable used for health education would describe how behaviour affects health. It would show what sort of behaviour promotes health and what is harmful. The fable should also give reasons for choosing healthy behaviour. By the end of the fable the sorts of behaviour that are best for health should be clear to everyone.

A sample health education fable

Here is a sample fable that was made up to show children the importance of cleaning their teeth regularly. The characters are a horse and a dog. When you make up your own fables, use animals that children in your community will recognize.

The horse and the dog usually ate their food together in the evening after a hard day's work. After the meal the horse would go to sleep straight away because he was tired. The dog was tired too, but he always cleaned his teeth before he slept. One evening the horse asked the dog, 'Why are you always cleaning your teeth? Why don't you sleep early like me so you will be rested for tomorrow's work?' The dog answered 'Cleaning my teeth makes them stronger. Dogs must have strong teeth for chewing bones and for protecting the house against dangerous animals.' The horse just laughed and went to sleep as usual.

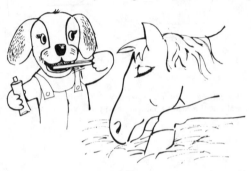

One day a friend brought the horse some crisp, hard apples. The horse loved apples and decided to save them until after dinner. That night while the dog was chewing his bones, the horse started to eat his apples. He took one bite of the hard apple, but just as he bit, he heard a loud crack. He felt a terrible pain in his tooth, and started to cry.

The dog ran to see what had happened to him. There on the ground next to the apple was a large piece of one of the horse's teeth. The horse cried 'Can't you put the tooth back? I want my teeth to be strong again.' Unfortunately it was too late. The dog couldn't help his friend replace the tooth.

After telling this fable, a health worker should ask children questions like: Why did the horse's tooth fall out? Why were the dog's teeth strong enough to chew bones? Do you want to be like the horse or the dog? What can you do to make sure your teeth stay strong?

Children could be encouraged to draw a picture like the one above to help them remember what they have learned.

What fables do you remember being told as a child? What are some of the common fables told in the community where you work? Are any of these related to health matters?

Talk to elderly people in the community to learn more local fables. Try to make up your own health education fables about the common health problems of children in your community. First tell the fables to a few children to see if they understand the main point. This is pre-testing. After making corrections, you can use the fable in your health education programmes.

Stories

Stories often tell about the deeds of famous heroes or of people who lived in the village long ago. An older person, instead of directly criticizing the behaviour of a youth, may tell a story to make his point. He may start by saying, 'I remember some years ago there was a young man just about your age . . . ' and then continue to describe what this young man did that caused trouble. Stories may also be a way of re-telling interesting events that happened in a village. So stories can entertain, teach history, spread news and information, and also serve as lessons about behaviour.

Purpose

Stories can be used to give information and ideas, to encourage people to look at their attitudes and values, and to help people decide how to solve their problems.

Group size

Stories can be told to individuals or to small and large groups. They also can be used on the radio to reach communities, regions or even whole countries.

Characteristics of a good story

The story should be believable. The people in the story should have names. They should do the kind of work that people in your community do. Their actions should be normal, not strange. Be sure that you do not name or describe real people in your story. If they hear the story they may become embarrassed or angry. The story should be short, otherwise people will become bored. They may also forget parts of the story. Five to ten minutes is all you need.

The story should make a clear point in the end. It should be obvious to the listeners which action is good and which is not.

Avoid scornful and unkind words in the story. If you say, 'This foolish mother did not bring her child to the clinic in time' some mothers may get angry. They too may have been unable to bring their child to the clinic on time. They may not listen to you again. Simply describe the actions of the people in the story. Let the listeners make up their own minds. If you tell the story well, the listeners will be able to judge correctly.

Always follow a story with discussion and questions. Do not tell the listeners which person in the story did the best thing. Ask the listeners for their own opinions. By encouraging people to think about the story and to discuss the points that impressed them, you will help them to learn more.

A sample story

Mrs Alto is a busy woman, but she always tries to do the best for her children. She is a seamstress. She uses the money she makes to buy good food and other things for her children. Last year she bought mosquito nets for her children. Now they sleep peacefully at night. Since fewer mosquitos bite them, the children do not get fever as often as they did before. As a result the children, and parents, are much happier.

Mrs Alto's son David is a bright boy. He always does well in school and this makes his parents proud. David has many friends. Thomas is his best friend.

One day Mr and Mrs Alto received a letter from their home town. Mr Alto's mother was very sick and the family wanted Mr Alto and his wife to come home right away. David asked if he could stay with Thomas while his parents were gone. Thomas' parents, Mr and Mrs Bella, agreed.

After staying for some days with Thomas, David could see that Mrs Bella was not like his own mother. Mrs Bella had a shop in the market. She stayed there very late in the evenings. Many times she gave the boys only a small amount of money to go out and buy rice and beans for their supper.

Thomas did not have a mosquito net. At night he and David would toss and turn because of the mosquito bites. They were always tired in the morning. One day David felt hot. Then he felt cold and had pains. He could not go to school for several days. The Altos returned to find David still sick. Mrs Alto took him to the health centre. When David recovered, he thanked his mother and asked her to talk to Mrs Bella about taking better care of Thomas.

Here are some questions for discussion. Why did David get fever? Why does David do well in school? How can a mother spend the money she earns to ensure that her children stay healthy? What advice should Mrs Alto give to Mrs Bella? How can Mrs Alto give the advice so that Mrs Bella will not feel hurt and angry?

If malaria is a common problem in your area, tell this story to mothers in your community. Change the names or occupations to make the story more relevant to the people. Now make up your own stories about health problems that are common in your area.

Case studies

In a way case studies are like stories except that case studies are real-life experiences. They are based on facts and present events as they really happened. Details of how to write and use a case study, and a sample case study are given in Chapter 5, pages 147–152.

Demonstrations

Demonstrations are a pleasant way to share knowledge and skills. They involve a mix of theoretical teaching and practical work that makes them lively. For details of how to plan and hold a demonstration, or series of demonstrations, see Chapter 5, pages 144–147.

Posters

A poster is a large sheet of paper, often about 60 cm wide by 90 cm high with words and pictures or symbols that put across a message. Posters are widely used by commercial firms for advertising products, and to reinforce the message being delivered by other mass media.

Purpose

Posters can be used effectively for three purposes.

- To give information and advice.

- To give directions and instructions.

- To announce important events and programmes.

Group size

The target group can be small or large. It can be the whole community. Sometimes you may also want to use posters with individuals. You may be counselling someone in the clinic, in the school, or at your office. If there are posters on the walls that relate to your client's problem, you may take the client to see those posters.

Content

A number of rules should be followed in making posters.

- All words should be in the local language.

- Words should be few and simple.

- Symbols that illiterate people will also understand should be used.

- Colour should be used to attract attention.

- Only put one idea on a poster. Too many ideas will make the poster look clumsy and confuse people. If you have several ideas to pass on, use a flipchart (see pages 222–225).

Posters announcing events should contain the following information.

- The name of the event.

- The date and time.

- The place.

- The organization sponsoring the event.

The poster should be big enough for people to see clearly. If you are using a poster with a group, make sure people at the back of the group can see it well.

Placing posters

Place posters where people will see them.

- Put them in places where many people are likely to pass (market areas, meeting halls).

- Ask permission before you put a poster on a house or building.

- Some places, buildings, rocks and even trees are sacred or special. Never put posters in these places. It may make people angry, and then they will not learn from your poster.

- Do not leave a poster up for more than one month. People will become bored and begin to ignore it. Change posters often to keep people interested. When you remove old posters, save them if they are in good condition. If a poster is worn and torn, dispose of it properly in a dustbin to set a good example.

Where to find posters

The ministries of health, education or information, voluntary agencies and some private companies may have ready-made posters to give or lend. Before you use such posters, pre-test them to make sure that they will be useful in your community.

You, and the people in the community, can design your own posters. A ministry or a private printer in town may be able to print them for you. Find out the cost of printing before you try this. The size of the poster and the number of colours affect the price. Ask the printer's advice about the cheapest way to design the poster. You may have to seek gifts of money to cover the cost. If the poster idea is very good, the ministry or a voluntary agency may decide to print it for nothing, but don't count on this. The community can make its own posters from local materials. The rest of this section describes how you can make your own simple posters, pre-test them and use them effectively.

Making posters

Materials that can be used include: large sheets of paper, pens, pencils, crayons, markers, paints and paint brushes, photos, old magazine pictures and glue.

Decide on how to use the poster. This will tell you how many to make. If you want to use the poster as an aid in your health

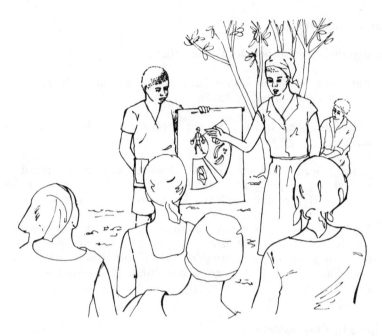

Posters can provide ideas and information. This health worker has attached the top of her poster to a wooden stick. This will make the poster last longer. Also she has asked someone from the audience to hold the poster so that she can point at the pictures and move about easily.

talks, you will need only one. If you plan to use it in the community, you will need many. First count the number of places in which you will put the posters. Do not make more posters than you need, because they will waste money.

Make a test drawing of the poster first, before putting it on a large sheet of paper. Involve your group or health committee in designing it. Make several copies so that you can pre-test the design before you make the final posters.

There are many ways to make pictures for your posters. You or someone else in the group or community may be able to draw or paint well. If there is no one who can draw, you can trace a picture from a book or magazine. Another way is to cut out pictures from old magazines and glue them on the poster. Photographs can be glued on too.

Involve people in making posters. Make one poster as an example and ask members of your committee to help you make more. Schoolchildren can help too. You might even hold a poster-making competition. This will interest people and help them learn more about health.

Pre-testing

Remember to pre-test your poster to be sure people understand and accept it. Posters cannot speak. If people do not understand a poster, they cannot ask it questions. All posters that you place around the village or town should have a very clear message.

Using posters in a group

If you are using posters with a group, attach the poster temporarily to a wall or tree in front of the group so they can all see. You may also ask for a volunteer from the group to help you hold up the poster. This may be better because the volunteer can walk around the group with the poster so everyone can see it closely.

Do not stand in front of the poster while you are talking about it. Do not try to hold it up yourself. This would make it much more difficult for you to communicate effectively with the group. Posters can be used as a basis for discussion. Do not hold up a poster and start explaining it right away. Instead:

- Ask everyone to look at the poster carefully. Give them a chance to see it well.

- Ask people what they see. What do they think is happening in the pictures? Let them think for themselves.

- If there are words on the poster, find out if someone can read. Ask him or her to read it for the group.

- Add your own ideas as the discussion continues.

- Turn to the poster again at the end of your discussion. Ask once more what people think is the message of the poster. Repeating and reviewing the message of a poster helps people remember.

Protecting and storing posters

It is a good idea to glue a piece of cardboard to the back of a poster, at least at the top. This will stop it tearing when it is held up for a group to see. Posters should be stored in one of these two ways.

- They may be kept flat inside a cupboard with a blank sheet of paper on top to stop them getting dusty.

- They may be rolled up with a string or rubber band around them. If you attach a small tag to the poster with the title and topic, then you can identify the poster without having to unroll it.

Be sure to keep posters dry and free from dust.

Displays

A display is an arrangement of real objects, models, pictures, posters, and other items which people can look at and learn from. Displays can be very simple or very sophisticated. They are most successful if they use a variety of materials to attract people. The illustration shows two displays using posters

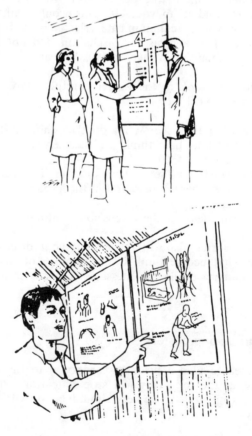

Displays range from very simple to highly sophisticated. They always use a variety of materials which make them attractive to people and facilitate learning.

Purpose

A display provides ideas and information, but whereas a poster contains only one idea, a display has many. The ideas usually relate to one theme such as 'Better farming methods' or 'How to build a poultry farm' or 'How your child develops and grows'.

Group size

Displays are usually set up where large numbers of people will pass by and see them. For example you may set up a display at a market or in the community hall. Everyone will be able to walk past one by one, or in small groups, to look at the display.

Materials

A display is made up of things that people can look at and learn from. You can use posters, photographs, real objects and models. You may have seen expensive displays, put up by companies or agencies, that use slide projectors and tape recordings. We are concerned here with simple displays you can make yourself.

Since posters and photographs are discussed in other sections of this chapter, we will only look in this section at how to prepare real objects and models.

Real objects

Real objects are just that—real. If your display is on 'Family Planning Methods', you would display real IUDs, pills, diaphragms, condoms, and foams. If your display is about 'Weaning Diet', you would show real foods and the tools used to prepare them, making sure that the food items do not spoil.

Models

You may have seen paper, cloth or plastic flowers that look like real flowers. They are models. Models might be used for three reasons.

- If the real object is not available, for example, certain fruits may be out of season or certain food items may spoil if left out on display. You can make models of such items.

- If the real object is too big to put on display. In this case you can make a small model. A lorry or a well, for example, would be too large to put on display.

- If the real object is too small to be seen easily you can make a larger model. For example, many insects are too small to be seen easily.

Models can be made of different materials. Clay, mud, wood, stone, straw, paper, cloth, and paper pulp (see below) are just some of the materials you can use for a model.

You must write on the display that the object is a model so that people will understand the display. Be sure to say if the model is larger or smaller than the real object. This will help people know

---

How to make paper pulp models

1. Tear old newspapers into small pieces about the size of your little finger-nail.

2. Soak the pieces in water in a pot (bucket or gourd) for one whole day.

3. Remove the pieces from the pot and squeeze out as much water as possible.

4. Mash the pieces of newspaper in a mortar with a pestle until they are completely mixed.

5. Dry the mashed material (pulp) in the sun until it is completely dry. Leave it on one side for the moment.

6. Make the basic shape (papaya, chicken, banana, etc) with wire, small sticks, wood strips, string or whatever is available. This will look like a skeleton of the thing you are making.

7. Wrap the shape in pieces of dry newspaper to make it look like the object you are making.

8. Prepare a smooth paste using water plus starch or wheat flour.

9. Put the dried paper pulp into a pot, then add some of the starch.

10. Mix the paper pulp and starch with a stick. Keep adding more starch bit by bit and stir until everything sticks together well. If the mixture is too dry or too watery it will not stick to the model.

11. Take some of the pulp mixture in your hand and mould it around the basic shape of the model that you made earlier until it looks like the object.

12. Tie string, straw or raffia to any part of the model. Hold the model by the string, and hang it up by the string to dry.

13. Paint the model with any available paints. Colours should be as much like the real thing as possible—don't make a blue banana!

---

what the real object is like. Here is an example of what you might write under a model of a mosquito in a display about malaria: 'Model of a malaria mosquito about 20 times larger than life-size.'

Help in making models can come from many people in the community. The carpenter and mason can help make small model houses, wells and latrines. Schoolchildren can help make model fruit and vegetables with clay and paper pulp. The tailor can help make small model clothes.

Setting up a display

Find out how much space you will have for your display items. Select your display items according to the space you have. Do not crowd too many things into a small space.

Find out what can be used to support your display. Will there be tables, benches, chairs, poles or walls? Choose your display materials according to this. If you only have wall space for a display, you may not be able to use large models or real objects. Instead, you could use photographs, posters and small objects.

Arrange all display materials in a logical order. Individual items might be numbered so people know what to look at first, second and so on. For example, if your display shows the steps needed to build a well, place each photo or model in order from left to right, or top to bottom. Place them in an order that is easy for people in your community to understand and follow.

Make sure all materials are securely fastened to the wall or table. You do not want your photos, posters, models or objects to fall down, blow away or be picked up by other people.

Make sure that there is a clear explanation for every item in the display. This may be in words, symbols or pictures. Displays, unlike demonstrations, are usually left alone. If there is not a clear explanation for the items, people will have no-one to ask for help in understanding the display.

Storing display items

You will probably want to use display items several times. Be sure to keep them in a dry place. Cover models to keep off dust. Insects may try to destroy models made from wood, cloth or paper pulp. If you do not have dry and insect-free storage for these items, it is better to make your models from clay and other strong materials.

Flipcharts

A flipchart is made up of a number of posters that are meant to be shown one after the other. In this way several steps or aspects of a central topic can be presented such as 'prevention of burns' or 'how to dress a small wound'. Flipcharts, with blank pieces of paper are also useful for recording ideas that come out of group meetings or discussions.

Purpose

To give information and instructions, or record information.

Group size

Flipcharts are best used with small groups. They are not put up around the community like posters.

Where to find flipcharts

You may get flipcharts from your ministry or voluntary agency, but it is usually best to make your own. Making your own has the advantage that the topics you include will exactly match the educational needs of the group and community.

Making flipcharts

The individual posters or charts are joined together at the top. You can probably think of many ways to do this—glue, string, or nailing or tacking posters to a long, thin piece of wood. Since the individual charts will be turned over many times, join them with something that will stop them tearing or coming apart. If you have the resources, you can cut a thin piece of wood the exact size of the posters, and glue or tack all the posters together at the top of this board. You can then stand the board on a chair. This will make it easier for you to show the flipchart and turn each poster, one after the other.

A flipchart tells a story. On each chart or poster one idea is presented. The illustrations are arranged in order to match your talk or story. Five is a good number of posters to put in a flipchart, although you may have more or less. If you have too many ideas, people may not remember everything.

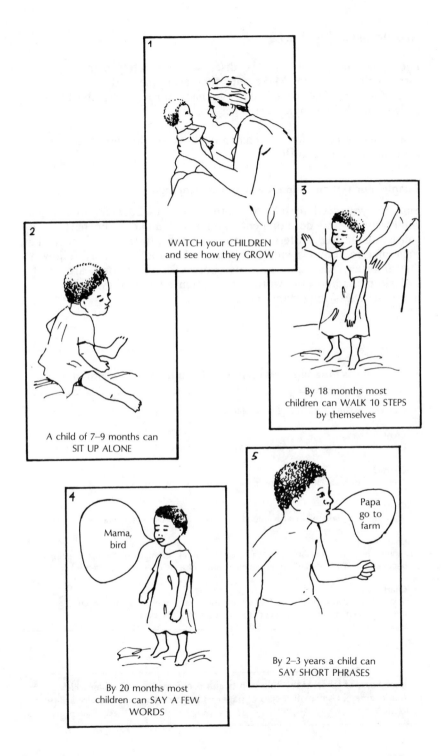

WATCH your CHILDREN
and see how they GROW

A child of 7–9 months can
SIT UP ALONE

By 18 months most
children can WALK 10 STEPS
by themselves

By 20 months most
children can SAY A FEW
WORDS

By 2–3 years a child can
SAY SHORT PHRASES

Mama,
bird

Papa
go to
farm

How to use a flipchart

Each chart or poster must be discussed completely before you turn to the next one. Make sure that everyone understands properly each idea. At the end, go back through the charts to review and help people remember the ideas.

You can get ideas for the charts by looking through books and magazines about health.

Sample flipchart on child growth and development

Suppose you need to talk to mothers of preschool children about child growth and development. You could make a flipchart consisting of five posters, as shown in the illustration. Notice that each picture shows a single, separate idea and that they follow a logical order. Also notice words chosen for the posters are short and simple. Important words are written so that they stand out more than less important ones.

Ideas for a flipchart on preventing blindness in children

Can you make up pictures and simple words for the five charts?

Chart 1
Eyes are important to our children. We must protect them.

Chart 2
Keeping flies away from children's eyes helps prevent blindness.

Chart 3
Washing face well, especially around the eyes, helps prevent blindness.

Chart 4
Eating fruits and vegetables that are red (tomatoes, oranges, oil from red palm fruit, papaya, carrots) and dark green spinach and other leafy greens prevents blindness.

Chart 5
Measles can cause blindness. Prevent measles with immunization. If a child gets measles, keep him in a darkened room to protect his eyes.

Now think of some of the common health problems in your village. Pick one example. Use small pieces of paper as practice sheets and make a flipchart.

224

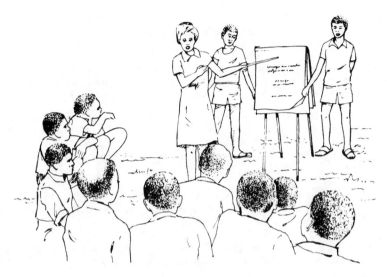

This health worker is using a small easel or stand to hold her flip-chart. This keeps the chart steady and makes it easier for the whole group to see. She has also involved members of the group in helping her with the programme.

Flannelgraphs

A flannelgraph is a board covered with flannel cloth. Pictures and words can be placed on the board to reinforce or illustrate your message. When you prepare a talk that you want to illustrate you should think of the different pictures, words and shapes you will need for the topic.

Purpose

Flannelgraphs help people see more clearly what you are saying during a talk.

Group size

Flannelgraphs are used mostly with small groups. Like posters, flannelgraphs must be seen clearly by everyone. In a large group this would be difficult. If you have an office, you can keep the flannelgraph there, to use with individuals who come for help.

225

Making a flannelgraph

If you want a flannelgraph, you will probably need to make your own. There are two basic parts to a flannelgraph. One is the cloth-covered board. The other is a set of pictures which you can stick to the board.

1. First make a board. Cut a square or rectangular piece of wood that is less than one metre long. The width can be shorter than the length.

2. Buy three metres of thick, coarse cloth. Thin, slippery cloth will not work.

3. Put one metre of cloth over one side of the board. If the cloth has a rough side and a smooth side, the rough side should be on the outside. Save the rest of the cloth.

4. Fold the edges of the cloth around the board. Fix the edges securely to the back of the board with nails, tacks or glue.

5. At this point you should have a board with its front covered with cloth.

6. Now you need pictures to stick on the board.

7. You can cut pictures from magazines or draw your own. Look for pictures of single subjects such as a person, a baby, a type of food, a vehicle, a tree, and so on.

8. The picture should be about as big as your hand. If the picture is too small, no one will see it.

9. You can also cut out words that are in large print. Words such as family, health, food, danger, help, and prevent can be put on the chart along with the pictures.

10. Cut out the pictures and words. Leave a border around them about as wide as your smallest finger-nail.

11. Now paste the pictures and words onto the rest of the cloth. If the cloth has a smooth side, stick the pictures on that side. If you do not have paste or glue you can make some with starch, or wheat flour, and water. Smooth out the pictures on the cloth with a slow sweeping motion of your hand.

12. Cut out the picture carefully, with its cloth backing. This time trim off the small border.

13. Allow the paste to dry before using the pictures. Otherwise they may get detached from the cloth.

14. Try to place your pictures on the board. You will see that the rough cloth on the back of your pictures and words sticks to the rough

cloth on the board. Now your pictures will stay on the board while you talk.

15. If you can find, or buy, small pieces of different coloured rough cloth, you can cut out different shapes. The shapes of perhaps fruit, plants, animals or buildings, can be stuck on the flannelgraph just like pictures.

16. You can also paste pictures on the smooth side of sandpaper. The rough side of the sandpaper will stick to your flannelgraph.

How to use a flannelgraph

Put the flannelgraph on a table, chair or easel.

Place all the pictures, words, and shapes you will need on a table near the flannelgraph so that you can see them and reach them easily. Carefully place the pieces in the order in which you will use them.

While you talk, place pieces on the board, or remove them from the board, as you make your points. Be careful not to turn your back to the audience. Practise working sideways.

You may want to arrange several pieces to make a whole picture. This may actually look like a poster. Be careful where you put the pieces. If you put a chicken on top of a man's head, or something funny like that, people will laugh and not concentrate on the message.

Encourage participation. When you make a point, ask someone from the group to come up and select the right piece and place it on the board. During the review at the end of your talk ask members of the group to use the flannelgraph to make their own points.

Storing the flannelgraph

The flannel-covered board itself should be kept dry and covered. If it gets wet or dusty, it will not hold the pieces very well. Keep your pictures, words and shapes in envelopes or paper bags. Write on the outside of the envelope or bag what pieces it contains. An envelope may be marked, for example, 'vegetables' or 'animals'. Another way is to put all the pieces for a particular programme in one bag. The next time you want to give the same talk, you will be able to find all the pieces easily. Write the title of the programme on the envelope.

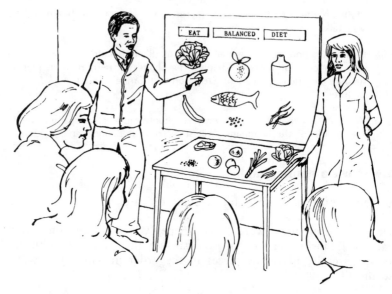

Participation is possible with a flannelgraph. Members of the audience can come up and select pictures and words to put on the cloth-covered board. In this way, they show their own ideas about the problem being discussed.

Photographs

Photographs are a useful educational tool. They can show situations and objects exactly as they are in reality. But people have to be used to looking at photographs to be able to understand what they represent.

Purpose

Photographs can show people new ideas. They can also show new skills being practised. Show and discuss them as you would show a poster or a flipchart. They can also be used to support and encourage new behaviour.

Group size

Photos are best used with individuals and small groups. This is because of their size. It is expensive to make large photogrphs. Still, they have to be big enough to be seen. A photograph about the same size as a page in this book, or a little larger, is about right. Photographs can sometimes be pasted together to form posters for the whole village to see.

Where to find photographs

The cheapest way to get photographs is to cut them out of magazines. Sometimes ministries and voluntary agencies have files of photographs. They may give you copies of these to be used in health programmes.

You may hire a commercial photographer to take photos for your programme. Black and white photos are the cheapest and are quite suitable for most purposes. In fact, in most small towns, photographers only make black and white photos.

Content of photographs

Several points need to be kept in mind when you choose photographs.

- The people and surroundings in a photograph should look similar to the people who will look at the photograph. People may not understand the idea in the photo if it looks strange to them.

- The photo should focus on one clear idea. Close-up photos are usually better than ones showing wide areas. If the photo shows too many things happening, people may not be able to see the main point.

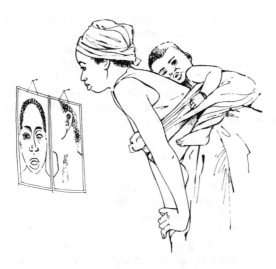

These photographs are well chosen for health education. They are familiar to the woman looking at them, and they each show one clear idea.

- A series of photographs can be used to show different scenes in a story. They could also show the steps needed to complete a project or to practise a skill.

- Community events such as plays and clean-up campaigns are good subjects for photographs. You may request a photographer from the ministry or get gifts of money to pay for a local photographer to attend the events. People will feel proud when they see themselves in the photos, and they will be encouraged to continue their good work. Such photos should be posted on the wall of the school, at the health centre or in the community hall. Praise and interest will support people's changes and improvements.

Storing photographs

After long use, photographs may become worn at the edges or torn. Your photographs will last longer if you can tape or paste them on to strong cardboard.

Make sure your photos do not get wet. Keep them in a file or box in a dry place. Organize your photo files according to the topic or subject of the photos.

Projected materials

Projected materials are simply educational materials that are shown to people using a projector. Projectors are machines that can only be used where there is electricity, and an experienced person to operate them. They need to be well cared for by someone who knows how to repair them if something goes wrong. Although these drawbacks mean that projectors are not usually practical for the community health worker to use in his or her village, a brief introduction to their use is given.

Purpose

Projected materials are useful to underline the most important points in a talk or lecture. Therefore you should prepare your talk first. Then make or find transparencies or pictures that show the point well and help to clarify or illustrate it. Projected materials can also help people to learn a new skill, but a picture without practice sessions is not enough. Therefore, always include discussion or practice if you are using projected materials for teaching.

Group size

Projected materials are useful for groups of 30 people or less. If the group is too large, not everyone will be able to see. There are some small viewers for slides that can be used with one person.

Types of projectors

Overhead projectors

These machines show transparencies, which are clear, plastic sheets. You can write on them with special ink or wax markers and the writing can be rubbed out later.

You can make the transparencies in advance, or write on them during your talk, while they are on the projector. People usually prepare a series of sheets and use them like a flipchart. The use of projected drawings and words makes a lecture more interesting.

Slide projectors

Slides for this kind of projection are taken by camera. Instead of being printed, like photographs, the pictures are produced on small pieces of clear plastic, and usually mounted in cardboard frames to protect them. Although slides are small, the projector makes the picture appear large against a wall or screen.

Slides can also be shown in a series. Often special boxes can be attached to the projector to hold the slides and make it easy to show one quickly followed by another. A tape recorder with music and words can be played along with the slides. This seems

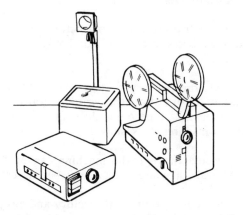

From left to right: slide projector, overhead projector, and film projector.

very much like a film or movie. In fact sometimes slides are joined together and called a film strip. Then you will need a film projector.

Check with different ministries and voluntary agencies to find out what slide programmes and film strips they have. Some topics may be relevant to your work. Always look at the programme before you show it to others. Make sure it is right for your community.

Opaque projectors

With an opaque projector you do not have to prepare special materials like slides or transparencies. This projector will show pictures, photographs, diagrams and words direct from a book, magazine or newspaper. It is not even necessary to cut these materials out.

If you are giving a talk you can find pictures that are related to your topic and show them. This will help the audience get a better idea of what you are talking about. The problem with this projector is that it is large and heavy. Modern slide and overhead projectors are lighter and easier to carry.

Where to find projectors

Even if you work with a ministry or agency that owns some of these machines, you may have difficulty getting one yourself. Projectors are usually available at your state, regional or national ministries. The ministries may loan you a machine for short periods and send someone to run it.

Using projected materials

- Five to ten good transparencies or pictures are enough for a talk. People may become confused and miss your points if you show too many.

- Each individual transparency or picture should be simple. If there is a lot of information the writing, drawing or pictures have to be small and it becomes difficult for the audience to see what the transparency is showing.

- Materials projected through the machine can be shown on a light-coloured wall, a white sheet or a special screen.

This is only a brief description of projectors and projected materials. If you would like to use them, you will need more skills. Find out if your ministry or agency gives demonstration classes on the use of these machines and on the preparation of materials for projection.

Tape recordings

The type of tape we are concerned about here is the cassette tape. These can be played on small, portable machines that use batteries.

Because of the expense of buying the machine, the tapes and the batteries, it is unlikely that this tool can be used by community health workers. Middle-level, for example district, and front-line, for example community, health staff, however, may find it useful as an aid in various circumstances.

Purpose

To provide health information and strengthen the health message.

Audience

The most common use of tapes is with groups. Sometimes in the clinic, hospital or school setting, individual patients or pupils can be requested to listen to a tape on a health topic related to their interest or problem.

Types of tape programmes

Lectures

Once a lecture has been recorded, it can be played whenever there is a group or an individual who wants to hear about the topic. To make the recording more lively and interesting, it is a good idea to play some music briefly at the beginning of the tape. The whole recording should be short, no more than 10 to 15 minutes. Since the audience has nothing to look at, they will become bored if the talk goes on for too long.

Radio programmes

These can be taped and played again for anyone who missed hearing them.

Role-playing and group discussions

When you play back the tape of a discussion or role-playing exercise, people can hear themselves. This will teach them about their behaviour, attitudes and values. Before recording a discussion or play, ask everyone if they agree to be recorded. It may surprise or embarrass some people if you record them without their knowledge. It is usually better to erase the tapes after the session. People may have said things that they do not want others outside the group to hear.

Statements from important people

Short recorded statements from important people can be used to liven up and reinforce your own lecture or health message. It also adds prestige and weight to the statement.

Tape with slides

Slides and tapes together make an interesting programme, but it needs to be planned carefully. The talk that you want to record on to the tape should be written out first. This is called the script. The script should be clearly marked to show exactly when to change the slides. The person operating the machine will read the script while the tape is playing, and change the slides at the right time.

Storing tapes

Many cassette tapes come in small plastic boxes when you buy them. It is necessary to keep the tapes in these boxes so that dust and dirt do not spoil them. If you do not have these small boxes, find a larger box or case for storing your tapes.

If you have a combined tape recorder and radio, do not leave the tape inside the machine while you are playing the radio (unless you are actually recording a radio programme). Tapes may pick up crackling sounds if left inside the machine. Also do not store tapes near other electrical machines, for the same reason. When you get your tape recorder, ask how to clean it so that it will not damage or put extra noises on the tapes.

Put a label on all educational tapes. The label should show the title of the topic, the name of the person or group speaking, and the date on which the tape was recorded. This will make it easier to find the tapes when you need to play them again.

Films or movies

People like films, because they provide action, colour and sound. They are a useful communication medium.

Purpose

Many different kinds of films are made. Some provide mainly information. They look like lectures that use sound and visual aids. Some demonstrate skills. Others are like plays, and show real-life situations. People can learn about new behaviour, attitudes and values in these films. Many are for entertainment.

Group size

Films can be shown to the whole community, but the larger the group, the less participation there will be. If possible, show films to groups of 30 people or less.

Where to find films

Ministries, libraries, voluntary agencies and some companies have films that can be borrowed. You will also have to borrow a film projector and possibly a small movie screen. Obviously you need electricity or a generator to show films. You may also need a skilled person to run the projector.

Choosing films

Do not base selection of a film only on the title. You should see the film first or talk to someone you trust who has seen it. Before you agree to show the film ask yourself these questions.

● Is the film in a language that the people understand?

● Does the film have correct and up-to-date information?

● Will the culture of the people in the film and the setting of the film look familiar to the people who watch the film?

● Does the film contain ideas that are practical for the community?

If the answer to any of these questions is 'no', do not choose that film.

You may think it is difficult to find a film for which the answer is 'yes' to all those questions. This is often true. Films are expensive to make. It is not possible to make a film to match the needs and culture of every community. It is often better to use plays, stories, puppets and demonstrations, because these can match your local culture.

Showing films

To have a good film show, you need to do the following things.

- Find a time and place that will be convenient for everyone who wants to watch.

- Pass the word around the community, neighbourhood or group so that many people will come.

- Show the film at night or in a place that can be darkened.

- Tell people, before showing the film, what it is about. This will help them know what they should look for and expect to learn.

- Make sure that everyone has a clear view of the screen. If too many people come and crowd the place, the view may be blocked. You may have to show the film twice so everyone has a chance to see it.

After showing the film hold a discussion session. Ask the audience questions about the film. Get them to ask you questions. Make sure they understand the film's message. If the group is large, break it up into smaller groups. Ask other health and community workers to help with the discussions in each of these sections.

Newspapers

Purpose

The main purpose of newspapers is to spread information. They print 'news', which usually consists of reports of events. They also include 'features', which are articles on a particular topic, and 'editorials', which express opinions about various subjects.

Health topics can fit into any of these categories. Health news might be a report of the launching of an immunization campaign, or a speech about health made by a well-known official. A health feature might be an article by a doctor about a certain disease or health practice. A health editorial might urge people to take part in a clean water programme.

Newspapers reach many people, very quickly. The press can play a very important part in increasing people's knowledge about health.

Size of group

Newspapers come in all sizes, from very large to very small. A major newspaper in a national capital or other big city may reach hundreds of thousands of people throughout an entire country. Many are printed daily on large modern presses and are mainly concerned with national and international news.

However, smaller cities and towns frequently have newspapers of their own, which may be printed once a week. These papers have a special interest in local news, and a health event in your community might receive attention in such a newspaper.

Finally, the idea of a newspaper can be reduced down to the community level. Some villages and urban neighbourhoods have 'wall newspapers'. These are like posters. They can be hand-made, in just a few copies, and posted on walls where people gather.

Using newspapers for health education

Newspapers can be used for health education in several different ways.

One way is to help your own professional growth. It is important for you to be aware of what is happening in health and community development. Newspaper articles are a good source of new ideas. For example, there may be a story on a successful community programme in another part of your country. You may wish to discuss it with your community leaders to see how it might be adapted to your own community.

Other valuable information might be a new or improved treatment of a certain disease, or a statement by a high official on the importance of health, which you can use to encourage participation. It is a responsibility of every health worker to be as well informed as possible. Newspapers can help you in this. Cut out and save interesting articles. You may be able to use them later on in your talks, discussions, or community meetings.

The second way in which newspapers are useful is as a way of sharing information with others. Even though many of the people you serve may not be able to read, there will be some who can. Often these are among the community leaders. They will appreciate your sharing information with them.

Newspaper articles are also useful for children in school. Health articles give excellent practice in reading. They may also stimulate young people's interest in a health topic. Remember that many school-age children play an important part in caring for their younger brothers and sisters, and that an enthusiastic youngster is often a very good educator of parents.

Writing your own news story

If an interesting health event is going to happen in your neighbourhood or village, you should consider writing a news article, and taking or sending it to the newspaper that serves your area. Of course it may not be printed. But if the event is unusual, and the story is well written, it will stand a good chance. Newspapers, especially local ones, often need new material.

Even if the story is not printed, the task of writing it is a very good exercise. It forces you to think about how to express your message in a few clear, understandable words. This in turn makes it necessary to decide what are the most important facts and ideas you wish to communicate. This discipline will help you to communicate your message more effectively through other means as well.

Study a few examples of local news stories. You will probably find that most of them have several commom characteristics. They are generally quite brief, with between 100 and 300 words. They use simple words, short sentences, and short paragraphs. They tell the reader the most interesting or important things first. They answer the questions who? what? when? and where? and then tell why and how if there is enough space. Some news stories tell about an event before it happens. Others report on it afterwards. Both kinds of report can be useful.

Now let's apply these general rules to a particular situation. A certain village is holding an immunization clinic and has invited a popular local orchestra to attract people to the clinic and entertain them when they are there. Your first idea might be to start by describing the target diseases and why it is important for children to be protected against them. But this would not be a news story. Get the unusual feature 'up front'.

'Mothers can get their children protected against four serious diseases, and listen to good music at the same time'.

This answers the question who, and catches people's attention. Now let's answer the other key questions in the next paragraph.

'The popular Colima Mariachi Band will perform at a Special Health Festival (what) to be held on Saturday, 20 July, from 1.00 pm to 6.00 pm (when) at the town square in Santa Barbara Village (where).

Now it is time to explain why. Name the diseases against which the immunizations will be offered. Tell why they are important. If possible use some simple statistics—newspaper editors like facts and numbers. Also, if possible, use a quotation. If the President or Minister of Health has made a statement on the importance of immunization, use part of it. If not, use a quotation from your local or district health officer.

This example was written to be used before the event. If you are reporting after the event, start with the most important thing that happened.

'More than 200 children were protected against four serious diseases at the Santa Barbara Special Health Festival on Saturday, 20 July'.

Now try this technique on a real or planned event in your community.

Making your own health 'newspaper'

Stories like the one just discussed can be used in your own neighbourhood or village, even if they are not printed in a formal newspaper. The 'wall newspaper' mentioned earlier is one way. Perhaps a teacher in your community school would like to have his or her students make a wall newspaper as a class project. Or a local artist can write out and illustrate the story. Of course, if you have access to a typewriter and an inexpensive way of reproducing copies you may wish to prepare a one- or two-page paper for special occasions, or even on a regular once-a-month basis.

Magazines

Magazines are another branch of the mass media with some uses in health education. They tend to be less accessible for the health worker than newspapers. They are generally intended for audiences in a very wide geographical area and are therefore less likely to be interested in local stories.

Many magazines do, however, carry useful information about health. Magazines written for women, for example, often have very important articles on child care, problems of pregnancy and maternal health, food and nutrition, etc. Even magazines intended principally for the entertainment of the general public sometimes carry health information.

Like newspapers, magazines can be an important source of continuing education for you as a health worker. In fact, magazine articles tend to be longer and more detailed than newspaper stories. Also, as with newspapers, such articles can obviously be shared with readers in your community and used as a basis for discussion.

From the health education angle, however, probably the outstanding feature of magazines is that they are a source of pictures. Magazine pictures are usually more numerous and often of better quality than those in newspapers. Many are in colour. Frequently you will find attractive and useful pictures even in magazines that have no articles on health, for example, pictures of healthy families, various foods, and many other things. These pictures can be used on posters and flannelgraphs, and in many other ways. Some magazines are devoted entirely to health. These are sometimes published by professional organizations, such as nurses' associations, or by ministries of health. They are especially valuable to you for your professional growth and for training programmes.

Radio

Of all the communication media, radio may now be the most effective for reaching very wide audiences with important messages. Certainly this is true in large parts of the developing world. Even in remote areas many farmers carry radios with them to the fields.

Purpose

Radio programmes serve many purposes. Some are purely for entertainment. They provide popular music and dramatized stories. Others are informational. There are several news broadcasts each

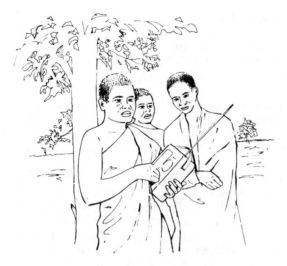

Even in the most remote rural areas, people often have radios.

day on most radio stations, at regularly scheduled times, and entertainment programmes may be interrupted for a news bulletin if something important happens. In addition, some radio programmes are designed for instruction or education. In many countries there are daily or weekly programmes on food and nutrition, on farming methods, and on health.

Finally, radio stations in many countries use very short messages, usually of one minute or less, for commercial advertising or to make public service announcements.

Coverage

The size of the area covered by a given radio programme or station varies widely. Some are national or even international. In some countries, all the radio programming is done at the national level, and the local stations in smaller cities outside the capital, if they exist at all, are used mainly as transmitters. In a number of other countries, however, there are local radio stations in smaller cities and towns. These may transmit national news and some other national programmes and also broadcast local news, local advertisements, and local educational programmes. So, even on the same radio station, some programmes may be designed for an audience of millions and others for the much smaller target of a district or region.

241

Use in health education

Health messages can be delivered by radio in many different forms. News items about health events can form a part of regular news broadcasts.

Special educational programmes on health topics can be broadcast, ranging in length from a few minutes to an hour or more. These can be in the form of talks, interviews, or discussion programmes at the radio station.

Because radio is a very important entertainment medium, some of the most effective messages can be delivered through songs, stories or plays. In many places there are very popular dramatic pro- grammes usually dealing with the problems faced by a family or group of individuals. When these problems are health-related, the message is contained in the way in which the characters deal with them. The audience does not realize that it is being educated as well as entertained, but it does receive the message, which is all the more likely to be remembered because of the form in which it is conveyed. Care needs to be taken with this method to avoid being over-emotional or trying to force people to change their views.

The information given in radio advertisements poses a special problem. Some of it is true, but some is only partially true, and some deliberately misleading. Many radio stations receive a large part of their financial support from the products they help to sell. When these products are harmful to health, as in the case of cigarettes, for example, the message that people hear is false. Part of your job is to help people to be aware of these things and to be careful listeners.

Radio meetings

It is usually possible to obtain a schedule of broadcasts in advance from the radio station that serves your area. This is important information for you. You can learn when programmes about health will be broadcast and what the subjects will be.

If you find out that a programme on a subject of importance to your community will be broadcast in a few days, spread the word. Put up notices in key places. Inform your health committee members and other community leaders. Urge everyone to listen. Better still, invite people to meet in a convenient place and listen together. Ask them to come a few minutes before the programme is scheduled to begin, so that you can introduce the topic. Then encourage discussion and questions as soon as the programme ends.

One of the so-called disadvantages of radio in health education is that it is a one-way medium. People cannot ask questions or talk back. By holding radio meetings, you can turn this disadvantage into an advantage.

One small word of caution: do not be afraid to say that you don't know. You will have prepared yourself as well as possible in advance of the programme. But something may be said that you do not fully understand, or some question may arise for which you do not have an answer. 'I don't know, but I will find out' is always an acceptable response, and is better than giving an answer that may not be accurate.

Getting your community programme on the radio

If you live within reach of a local radio station that does some of its own programming, you may be able to use radio more directly. Many local radio stations, like local newspapers, need interesting news items, interviews, or public service messages.

Radio news items, like those for newspapers, need to be brief; in fact, perhaps, even briefer than for newspapers. In the case of the story about the Santa Barbara Special Health Festival a radio news programme might use only the first two paragraphs, plus a list of the immunizations offered. But, unlike newspapers, radio stations may use the same item several times over a chosen period.

In many places radio interviews offer a special opportunity. If your community is having an important campaign or event, and especially if your health officer is well known and a good speaker, you could suggest to the radio station that they carry out a radio interview.

If this should happen, you would probably be expected to draft a list of suggested questions that will bring out the information you wish to convey. You will also need to be sure that your health officer or spokesperson gets to the radio station in good time, so that he or she and the announcer can get to know each other a little. You also need to be sure that the people of your community are gathered to listen.

Public service announcements

If you have access to a local radio station, it may be willing to broadcast very short public service announcements on health. These can serve many purposes. They may announce an event, like a health fair or immunization programme. Or they may give very brief health messages to serve as reminders to those who are listening.

Some announcements are as brief as 10 seconds. Even these can be useful, however, especially if they are broadcast many times. In a 10-second announcement you could say.

> 'It's Health Week in Santa Barbara. Remember, mothers: for your baby, breast milk is the best milk.'

Other public service announcements last 20, 30, or 60 seconds. Obviously you cannot include a very complicated message. But it is surprising how much you can say in a minute if you write the script carefully.

Try writing a few health messages of the various lengths just mentioned. This will be a good exercise in choosing the most important words and ideas, and seeing how many words you can fit into the given time.

Television

No other medium creates such lively interest as television. It can have a great impact on people. It can extend knowledge, influence public opinion, introduce new ways of life. In the health field, in urban areas and even in rural communities, it has already served as a powerful advocate of healthy behaviour in many instances. This is especially so when the health workers are able to integrate television programmes into their local activities, and to extend the impact of the medium through group discussions on the lines we have already discussed for radio programmes.

There is a new aspect of television that has much potential for health education. This is the use of video films. In some areas, video films are shown to small audiences by local groups. These groups may, or may not, have commercial interests. There are even places where series of films are projected throughout the day and people go to the show just as they would go to a cinema.

Do you know whether this approach is being used for health purposes in your community or in other communities? Do you think it has value for health education? What problems do you foresee?

Publications

It has often been said of health educators that 'all they do is give talks and hand out booklets'. We know that this criticism is exaggerated. But it must be admitted that, in many educational programmes, too much dependence is placed on distributing written materials in the form of booklets, pamphlets, or flyers without the necessary back-up in the hope that they will do the job alone.

Even with a highly literate audience, written material alone will rarely, if ever, lead to healthier behaviour. This is especially true if the literature is filled with technical terms and jargon understood only by professional health workers, or if the booklets are poorly illustrated, written in long, complicated sentences, and printed in small type. Unfortunately this describes a great many booklets that health educators distribute to the general public.

It is, of course, self-evident that such material is even less useful for audiences with limited reading ability. To depend upon booklets or pamphlets to do all, or even a major part, of a health education task is to invite failure.

Purpose

Nevertheless, written materials can serve a useful purpose in an educational programme. Written materials can achieve the following.

- They can remind individuals or families of a health message they have already learned in other ways. For example the importance of protecting children against a specific disease.

- They can provide additional information about a health problem or health practice for those who have a special interest in it.

- They can show the steps that must be followed in order to achieve a certain health goal, such as the way to mix the salt and sugar for the oral rehydration drink.

- They can share information with those who may not have received it in other ways.

Using written materials in the community

You, as a community health worker, probably do not have the facilities to produce your own written material, beyond simple posters, wall newspapers, or single-sheet flyers. Therefore your task is to select, from what is available, the material that is most appropriate to your community's needs, and to decide how to use it most effectively.

Selection requires, first, that you know what is available. Your regional or national health education office should be able to tell you about written material on a particular topic and perhaps send you samples. Other potential sources of useful booklets include voluntary associations, professional associations and commercial sources. International organizations like WHO and UNICEF have prepared pamphlets for communities on a number of subjects (see the Reading List on pages 260 and 261).

Once you know what written material exists and how it may be obtained, there are several questions you need to ask yourself before deciding to use a certain booklet.

- Is it written in a language and style that people in my community can understand?

- Is it well illustrated? Will the pictures seem familiar and relevant to my audience? This is a special problem in the case of pamphlets produced on an international scale. They may show houses, clothing, etc., that will seem alien and strange to your community, and this strangeness may interfere with the usefulness of the publication.

- Does the booklet contain the message I wish to convey? This is an especially important question in the case of commercially produced pamphlets. They may be very attractive and give useful information, but may also contain a hidden advertisement that is contrary to your purpose.

- Assuming that relatively few copies will be available, how can I make most effective use of them?

In general, booklets or pamphlets are best when they are brief, written in plain language, full of good pictures and, above all, when they are used to back-up, rather than form the basis of an educational programme.

Local or traditional media

In many countries health messages may be communicated through traditional media such as art, town criers, songs, plays, puppet shows and dance. These are discussed below.

Art

Shapes such as hearts, crosses or those of certain leaves have meanings for people. The meanings are different in different cultures. The use of animals in art also has meaning. An owl in one culture may mean wisdom, in another it may mean evil. Other animals are used as symbols to represent such character-istics as honesty, cleverness, laziness and courage.

Colours have meaning. A painter or weaver will choose colours for a purpose. Some colours are considered lucky. Some colours are thought to be best for children, some for adults. Meanings may range from bravery to cowardice, purity to evil. Some colours are used for special circumstances.

Talk with the weavers, painters, carvers, potters and other artists in your community. Find out the meaning of certain shapes, signs, animals, plants and colours. Use these symbols when you design a poster or other visual aids such as flipcharts, and flannelgraphs.

If you are designing a poster about the dangers of drinking untreated stream water, find out what signs, colours or animals mean danger. Use them on the poster. If you want a poster that shows the benefit of immunization, use colours and symbols that mean good luck and happiness. Your educational message will be clearer if you use traditional art forms and symbols.

Involve the traditional artists in your village in designing and making educational tools. The artists could go with you to a school to help teach the children about health and art at the same time. With the guidance of the traditional artists, children could do art projects with a health theme.

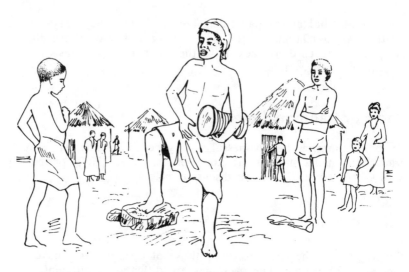

A town crier uses his voice, drums, and sometimes bells to spread important information throughout a community. Village leaders can use town criers to help communicate ideas and announcements concerning health.

Can you name all the artists in your community? What different kinds of art are there? We mentioned some that you can look at. How about art that you can hear? Poetry and music are two examples. Can you name others?

Do you have any examples of traditional art in your house? Do you know the meaning of the signs, shapes and objects on the piece of art? How could you use these in your educational programmes?

Town criers

Before radios and newspapers were invented, people had ways of spreading information and news. In many rural areas there are no newspapers, and radios only carry regional or national news. In most villages, then, there are still other ways of spreading the word about an important event or idea. Announcement by the town crier is one of these ways.

Purpose

If the leaders of a town or village want to get information to their community quickly, there are usually special people who can help them. These people have the job of spreading information. When they have something to say they may use a bell or drum to attract attention. Drum beats and other sounds can be a special code or signal that people understand.

Place

If the village is small, the town crier may go to a central place and begin announcing the message from the leaders. If the village is large, the town crier will walk around every section. In the larger towns, there may be several town criers to ensure that the news spreads quickly to all parts of the community. The announcements often sound like songs.

Methods

Town criers may use their own voices or various musical instruments, or both.

Content

The message carried by town criers could be to ask everyone to assemble at the chief's house, or at the town hall, for an important meeting. The message could be news from a neighbouring village. It could also be a warning about some danger like the outbreak of a disease. Town criers may announce the birth of a baby or the death of an elder.

Educational use

Many of the messages normally delivered by town criers relate to health. This is good, but you cannot go out singing messages yourself. People in the village know who is the real town crier and may only respect information coming from him or her. Nor can you ask the town crier to make the announcement for you. He or she works under the orders of the town leaders.

Therefore the way to involve town criers is through the town or village leaders, with whom you will probably already be working closely if you are planning a community health programme. The leaders can tell the town crier to help you. Here are examples of messages that could be passed on.

- A reminder to mothers to immunize their children.

- A request that people participate in a village clean-up campaign.

- A call for people to work on a community project such as digging a well.

- A warning about dirty water during a cholera outbreak.

Songs

People sing to express ideas and feelings. Many songs are about love and sadness. Songs may tell a story of a famous person or event. Some songs are religious, others are patriotic. Songs are sung to help children fall asleep or to celebrate special occasions. They can also help to educate people. Singing comes naturally in certain cultures, but not in others.

Purpose

Songs can be used to give people ideas about health. If the tune is attractive, people will remember the song and the information it contains.

Depending on the local culture, songs can be used at the beginning of a health talk, a meeting, or any other organized programme to create enthusiasm and interest. They can also make a meeting end on a happy note.

Size of group

The group can be large or small. Songs may also be played on the radio to reach a wider area and audience.

Plays

A play portrays life and people and tells a story that usually involves conflicts and emotions. The action and the dialogue are typically designed for theatrical performance with dramatic effects.

Purpose

Just like stories, plays make us look at our own behaviour, attitudes, beliefs and values in the light of what we are told or shown. Plays are especially interesting because you can both see and hear them. They can even be used to raise funds for community self-help and other projects.

Size of group

Plays are usually performed for large groups and are intended to reach whole communities.

Content

A play is based on a story. The story may be true, or it may seem like the truth. The story has a beginning and an end. The people who are putting on the play know the whole story, but the audience does not.

250

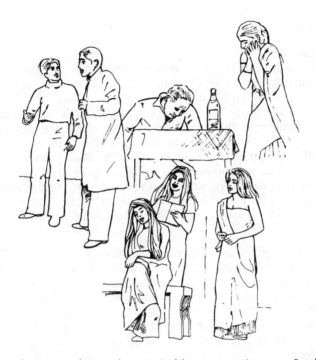

Here are three scenes from a play organized by a community group. People can learn about health through watching a play. This play is about a man who drinks too much alcohol. In each scene his family and friends try to find ways of helping him solve his problem.

A play has characters. That is people who act the different parts in the story. You can have any number of characters.

A play has scenes. If a story was acted out just as in real life, it could take several days. A play is generally a couple of hours long, but can be less. So, a play is made up of important short scenes or events.

A play can have a message. It may have a definite ending where all the problems are solved for better or worse. In this case, the lesson or message people learn from the play is usually obvious. Some plays have uncertain endings. They stop before the problems are solved. This makes the audience think hard. They wonder what might finally happen. They are curious about the characters. After this kind of play people like to talk and discuss. Since the message is not clear, people ask themselves 'What would I do next if I were that character?' This helps them practise decision-making skills.

Types of play

Traditional

In many cultures there are traditional plays that are performed during festivals and at special times of the year. They are often based on the lives and actions of ancestors, spirits, and famous people from the past. Traditional plays have a theme or message for the community. There may be ways in which the message relates to health. Such plays are closely tied to community values and beliefs. This makes people feel close to their culture and community when watching them. Social support grows out of this feeling. Traditional plays with health themes can be performed during a community health education programme. You may even write a play of your own resembling the traditional type.

Modern

You can write plays about present-day people. Take one of your health education stories and make it into a play. You could write out the words and actions for each character. To create more participation and interest, you could gather a small group of people who are willing to act in the play. Tell them the story. Let them choose what characters they want to be. Then ask the group to make up the speeches and action themselves on the basis of the story.

Materials needed

Clothes or costumes

What will the actors wear? They should wear the kind of clothes that would be natural for the characters they are playing. Farmers, businessmen, teachers, and religious people will all wear different kind of clothes. You might have to make special clothes for the actors to wear, but first see if they already have or can borrow suitable clothes.

Scenery

Where does the story take place: on a farm, in town, inside a house? You will want the audience to know. You may borrow furniture and you may paint large pictures on paper or wood. Do not spend a lot of money on scenery. Sometimes you can just tell the audience where the story takes place. Ask them to 'see' the scenery in their imagination.

Other materials

What kind of work do the different characters do: cooking, sewing, carpentry, farming? Collect or borrow things that these characters will need to use in the play so that they can look real while they act. A farmer may need a hoe or a knife. His wife may need cooking pots.

The actors

Find people in the community who are interested, who are not afraid to perform before an audience, and who can speak fluently. Schoolchildren can be successfully involved in plays as part of school health projects.

Announcements

You can make posters or use town criers to let people know about the time, place, and theme of the play. It is a good idea to give the play an interesting title. That way people will get an idea of what it is about. If it is a good title, people may come out of curiosity.

Planning the performance

The actors must practise until everyone knows his or her part in the play. You might ask some friends to watch practice sessions and give their comments. This is a way of pre-testing.

Make sure all materials needed are gathered together well in advance. Select a location for the play. If the play lasts longer than 30 minutes, people will need to be able to sit down. Plays can be done indoors or outside, depending on the weather. You can use a town hall, school, or other public meeting place. An audience can sit on a hillside, for example, for a play acted outside. In fact, you can do plays anywhere. Short plays can be performed in the market or the town square. People will gather when something interesting is happening.

Make sure that everyone can see and hear. You will probably want to repeat the play on several days if your village or neighbourhood is large. That way everyone will get a chance to see it.

Participation and learning

A play provides a good opportunity for people to participate. As we have seen, some can act, some can make or donate costumes and scenery, and others can make posters and announcements. Many different jobs go into making a successful team.

Everyone involved in putting on the play will learn because of their direct participation. They will learn the health messages of the play, and they will learn skills. These include planning and communication skills.

The audience will gain from watching the play, but you should make sure that they learn. Therefore, after the play, get the actors to discuss it with the audience. Questions can be asked back and forth to help the audience learn.

Puppets

Puppet shows are very similar to plays. The main difference is that puppets do the acting. People are still needed, however, to make the puppets move and talk.

Purpose

Just like stories and plays, puppet shows give examples of how people behave in real-life situations and can make us reflect on what is good and bad for health.

Uses of puppets

Puppets are made to look like small people or animals, but they behave like real people and become involved in a series of events resulting in conflicts and problems. Since you can make puppets look like animals, you can also use puppets to act out fables. You can even use a puppet to help you give a health talk.

Size of group

Since puppets are usually small, it is best to show them to relatively small groups—about 20 people. In that way, everyone is able to get close, and see what is happening. Of course, you can make puppets as large as children or as small as a mouse. Children usually love puppets. And their parents often enjoy watching with them. There are many types of puppet. Here are three common types.

Hand puppets

These puppets are made of cloth. You put your hand inside the puppet to make its arms and head move. You can hold hand puppets on your lap, or you can go behind a table and use the table as a stage for the puppets to stand on or you can make up a stage using a box and some cloth for curtains, as shown in the illustration.

String puppets

These puppets have strings tied to their arms, legs, head and mouth. You stand above the puppet and pull the strings to make it move. String puppets can be made of wood, cloth, cardboard, and other common materials. Local artists such as wood carvers can help you make puppets.

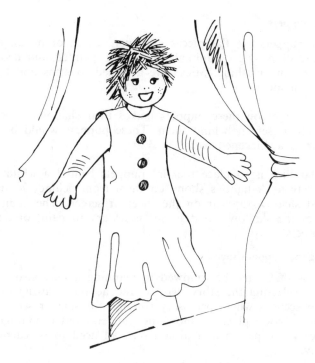

Hand puppets can be easily made, and used by children. Children can be encouraged to make up their own stories about health and act these out, using the puppets.

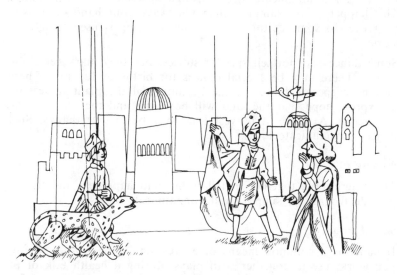

These are string puppets. Two or three people stand above and pull the strings to make the puppets move. As in a play, there are costumes and scenery.

Shadow puppets

Shadow puppets are flat pieces of paper, wood, or metal, made in the shape of people or animals. These are painted and decorated with faces and clothing. Sticks are attached to arms and legs to make them move.

Shining a light on these puppets makes their shadows appear large on a wall or screen behind them. These puppets would be used at night or in a darkened room.

A similar idea is to place the flat puppets behind a white sheet or a thin screen. A light is shone on them from behind, so that their enlarged shadows appear on the sheet or screen. The audience only sees the shadows so it is not necessary to paint or decorate the puppets.

Planning the puppet show

The steps that must be followed in planning a play also apply to puppets. Selecting the story, words, and action, drawing or painting scenery where necessary (though for smaller scenes), choosing a good place to show the puppets, and encouraging audience participation and discussions, all need to be carried out carefully.

Dance

People can communicate ideas through movement of their bodies. This happens, for example, when you wave your hand or wink your eye. In some cultures, traditional dancing is used to tell stories.

Some dances do not tell specific stories, but they mark certain events. There may be special dances for births or funerals. There may be a special dance for the beginning of the planting season to express hope that the land will be fertile and the crops productive. A dance at harvest time may be to give thanks. Such dances communicate ideas.

Purpose

To bring people together in fellowship and happiness and to provide feelings of support and communicate ideas.

Size of group

If dance is a common means of expression in the culture where you work, use it, together with plays, during a health talk or at a club meeting to communicate appropriate ideas and feelings of support.

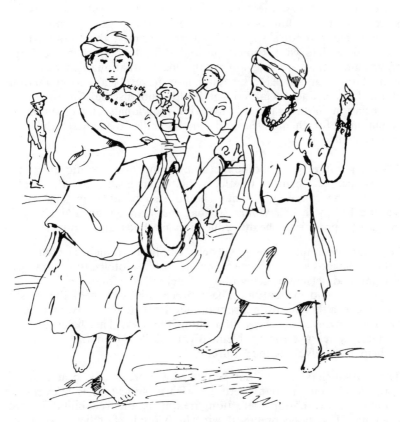

Dancing and music are traditional ways of communicating ideas. The movements of the hands and body convey a message to those who watch. Traditional ways of communicating can be used to convey health messages also.

Summary

The spirit of primary health care and the principles of health education call for community self-reliance in health development. Health education programmes must accordingly be designed with active community involvement. This will ensure that programmes reflect local realities, meet local needs, and use local resources. Since it would be unproductive to develop a health education manual that promotes standardized programmes, this manual has provided readers with knowledge and skills to help them develop programmes that are relevant to the local situation. Having studied the manual readers should now have (1) an understanding of the human and social side of health and disease; (2) an appreciation of the value of involving individuals and communities in planning for themselves, and (3) the skills to facilitate this involvement.

At this point readers should be able to mention specific examples of how people's behaviour effects their own health and the health status of the community. They should also be able to detect the reasons for these behaviours so that they can design and apply the most appropriate health education methods and strategies.

Important planning steps have been emphasized such as community diagnosis, objective setting, resource mobilization, strategy and method selection, scheduling of activities, monitoring of progress and evaluation. These procedures will yield the most effective health education programmes when community members are fully involved in every step along the way. This helps the community learn basic problem-solving skills which they can use to help themselves in the future.

The manual has shown that health education can be practised at many levels and in many settings. Health education is relevant for promotion, prevention, detection, treatment and rehabilitation programmes. It can be practised with individuals, families, groups and communities. Health workers themselves may also need education to improve the way they serve the public.

Health education should not be limited to any particular setting. Attention must focus on schools, social organizations, clinics, worksites and the community at large. People in each of these settings will have special needs which health education can address.

Another important issue raised in this manual is that health education consists of a wide variety of strategies and methods.

This is because health problems have many possible causes. Public awareness strategies help increase health knowledge. Community organization helps people acquire basic health resources. Social support strategies draw on the encouragement of family and friends to reinforce healthy action. A mixture of strategies is usually desirable. Although the choice of strategies may vary from problem to problem and from community to community, they all follow the basic ideal that health education should improve people's ability to make decisions and take actions to solve their own problems.

Finally, it should be emphasized again that the readers must feel free to adapt this manual to suit the needs of their countries. Already the provisional draft version has been translated into other languages in some countries in which it has been tested. The manual will be useful in training programmes and as a handbook for practitioners. Therefore the examples, stories, pictures and choice of words should be changed to fit the local social, cultural and organizational environment. If this manual is able to encourage readers to develop their own unique health education programmes, then it will have achieved its purpose.

Reading List

Alma-Ata 1978: primary health care. Geneva, World Health Organization, 1978 ("Health for All" Series, No. 1).

Community involvement in primary health care. Report of a workshop held in Kintampo, Ghana, 3-14 July 1978. Geneva, World Health Organization, 1979.[1]

Global strategy for health for all by the year 2000. Geneva, World Health Organization, 1981 ("Health for All" Series, No 3).

Health programme evaluation: guiding principles. Geneva, World Health Organization, 1981 ("Health for All" Series, No. 6).

OFUSU-AMAAH, V. *National experience in the use of community health workers: a review of current issues and problems.* Geneva, World Health Organization, 1983 (WHO Offset Publication, No. 71).

MCMAHON, R. ET AL. *On being in charge: a guide for middle-level management in primary health care.* Geneva, World Health Organization, 1980.

The community health worker. Geneva, World Health Organization, 1987.

UNDP/WORLD BANK. *Methods for gathering socio-cultural data for water supply and sanitation projects:* TAG Technical Note No. 1, Washington, The World Bank, 1983.[1]

UNICEF/WHO Joint study on water supply and sanitation component of primary health care, Geneva, 1979 (document JC22/UNICEF/WHO/79.3).[1]

UNICEF/WHO *Primary health care: the community health worker.* Report on a UNICEF/WHO Inter-regional Study and Workshop (Kingston, Jamaica) 1979/1980 (document PHC/80.2).[1]

UNICEF/WHO JOINT COMMITTEE ON HEALTH POLICY. *Community involvement in primary health care: a study of the process of community motivation and continued participation.* Report for the UNICEF/WHO Joint Committee on Health Policy, Geneva, 1977 (document JC21/UNICEF-WHO/77.2).[1]

WERNER, D. & BOWER, B. *Helping health workers learn.* Palo Alto, California, The Hesperian Foundation, 1982.

WHO Eastern Mediterranean Regional Office. Health education with special reference to the primary health care approach. *International journal of health education,* 1978, **21**(2) supplement.

WHO/TDR. *Community participation in tropical disease control: social and economic research issues.* Geneva, World Health Organization, 1983 (document TDR/SER-SWG(4)/CP/83.3).[2]

WHO Technical Report Series, No. 89, 1954 (*Health education of the public: first report of the Expert Committee*).

---

[1] Copies of these documents are available from: Division of Public Information and Education for Health, World Health Organization, 1211 Geneva 27, Switzerland.
[2] Copies of this document are available from: Special Programme for Research and Training in Tropical Diseases, World Health Organization, 1211 Geneva 27, Switzerland.

WHO Technical Report Series, No. 633, 1979 (*Training and utilization of auxiliary personnel for rural health teams in developing countries*).

WHO Technical Report Series, No. 690, 1983 (*New approaches to health education in primary health care:* report of an Expert Committee).

WHYTE, A. *Guidelines for planning community participation in water and sanitation projects.* Geneva, World Health Organization, 1986 (WHO Offset Publication, No. 96).